# MINDFULNESS
## and SLEEP

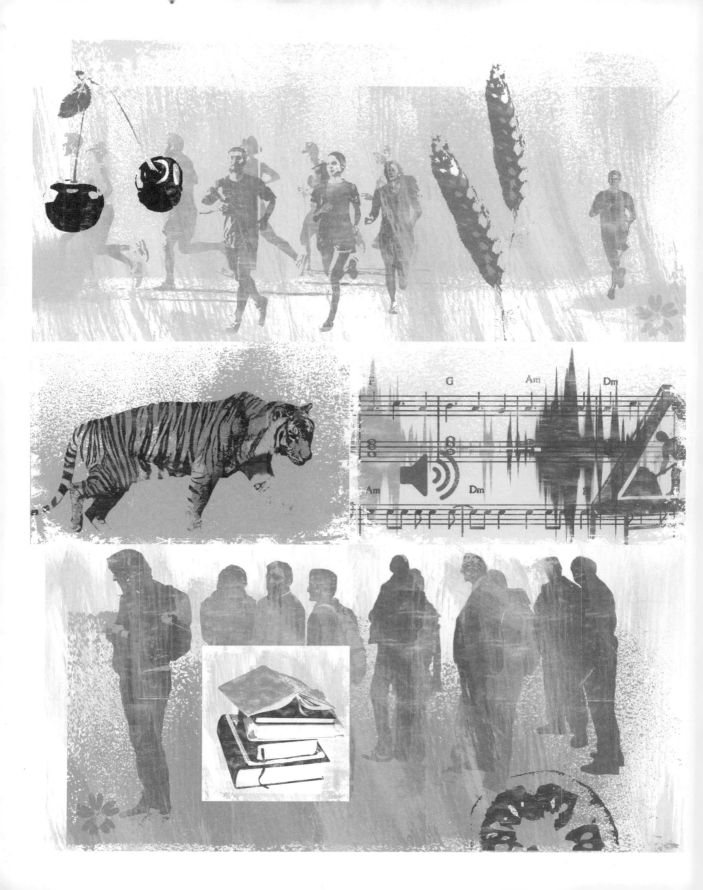

# MINDFULNESS
## and SLEEP

How to improve your sleep quality
through practicing mindfulness

## Anna Black

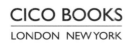

CICO BOOKS

LONDON  NEW YORK

FOR PIP—AWAKE ON THE OTHER SIDE
OF THE WORLD

Published in 2018 by CICO Books
An imprint of Ryland Peters & Small Ltd
20–21 Jockey's Fields      341 E 116th St
London WC1R 4BW      New York, NY 10029

www.rylandpeters.com

10 9 8 7 6 5 4 3 2 1

A CIP catalog record for this book is available from
the Library of Congress and the British Library.

ISBN: 978-1-78249-560-4

Printed in China

Editor: Rosie Fairhead
Designer: Emily Breen
Illustrator: Clare Nicholas

Commissioning editor: Kristine Pidkameny
Senior editor: Carmel Edmonds
Art director: Sally Powell
Production manager: Gordana Simakovic
Publishing manager: Penny Craig
Publisher: Cindy Richards

**Please note:** If you are having a sustained period
of difficulty sleeping, you should always visit your
physician for advice.

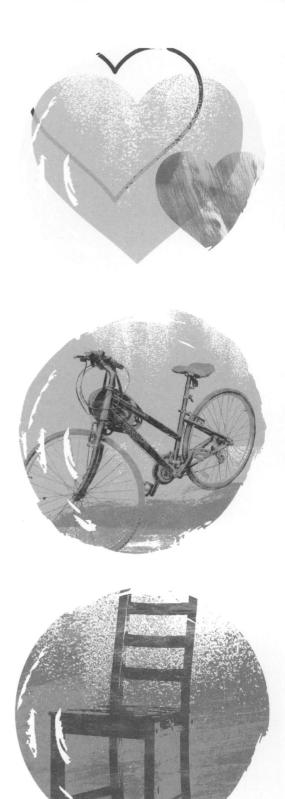

# CONTENTS

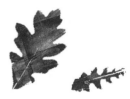

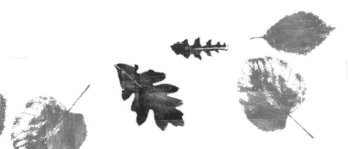

# INTRODUCTION

**Most people will at some point experience periods when they find it difficult to sleep. It is most often triggered by a stressful event, but it can also be caused by illness, whether physical or psychological. While some illnesses can cause insomnia, sleep and the physiological functions of the body are so intertwined that many medical conditions can also be exacerbated by, or be a result of, sleep deprivation.**

I was always someone who fell asleep within minutes of putting my head on the pillow. If I did wake in the night it was for so brief a time that it didn't affect my sleep quality negatively. I would sympathize with those friends who recounted tales of troubled nights,

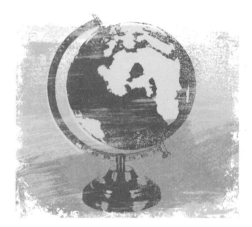

but I had no real understanding of how debilitating broken nights and sleep deprivation can be. Then everything changed. A combination of hitting my late forties and undertaking stressful building works on my home meant that I joined the millions who have trouble sleeping. And it is millions.

When I first started experiencing problems sleeping, I became interested in what was happening. Sometimes I would struggle to fall asleep as I found myself reviewing the latest building dramas of the day, and it would take an hour or two for me to fall asleep. At other times, I fell asleep quickly but then woke up because I was too hot (the night sweats of the menopause kicking in), and once awake I found myself thinking—and quickly became caught up in a spiral of "what if" and "if only" thoughts accompanied by physical feelings of tension in my shoulders and neck, and a sick sensation in the pit of my stomach. As well as thinking about what went on during the day, I would worry about why I wasn't asleep yet, totting up how many hours I already had slept (or not) and trying to guess how it would affect me the next day. I was now very much awake, and it would be a couple of hours before I would fall asleep again, often just before my alarm sounded. The common thread was always "thinking." My thoughts would keep me in a state of alertness—mentally and physically—that was the opposite of the sleep state.

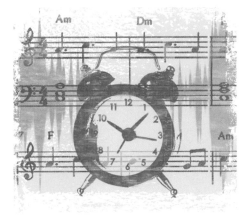

I began to pay attention to what happened. I noticed that if I caught myself hovering around that moment of awakening, I could sometimes lull myself back to sleep by repeating "not thinking, sleeping" to myself as a form of mantra. To catch that moment was tricky, though. I knew from my mindfulness practice how turning my attention to the body is particularly helpful when I am caught up in a cycle of negative thinking. Although there is a meditation practice called the Body Scan, which focuses the attention on the body (see page 68), I didn't want to get into the habit of doing that in order to fall asleep, so I started listening to a guided Yoga Nidra practice. Yoga Nidra is a meditation that is designed to promote deep rest and relaxation, and it became my go-to practice. I would do it when I went to bed and also in the middle of the night when I woke up. Sometimes I fell asleep during it, but at other times I was still awake at the end and that was okay. Even if I was awake I felt calm, relaxed, and rested. Realizing that I could achieve this despite being awake stopped me feeling the pressure to fall asleep. My whole relationship with sleeping shifted and

## What is Yoga Nidra?

Yoga Nidra is a traditional yoga practice designed to induce relaxation—physically, mentally, and emotionally. It has been described as "deep relaxation with inner awareness" (Swami Satyananda Saraswati, *Yoga Nidra*, 1976). Yoga Nidra is a systematic practice, usually between 20 and 50 minutes long, that involves first setting an intention or resolve before scanning through different body parts, followed by awareness of breath, feelings, and emotions, and a visualization. In order to relax fully, it is best done following guided instructions. As with the Body Scan on page 68, the intention is not to fall asleep. Many versions are available online, in apps, and as CDs, and I recommend exploring and finding one you like in terms of duration, content, and voice.

I found myself welcoming those awake times as an opportunity to practice. I probably wasn't getting any more sleep during this time, but the lack didn't feel so depleting, so overall I felt as if I was getting enough good-quality rest. What I was experiencing is supported by the research into mindfulness and sleep (see page 53).

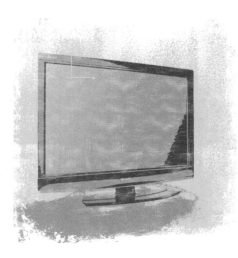

As well as noticing what happened during the night, I also started paying attention to what I was doing in the hours before bedtime. I noticed that those times I had a glass of red wine or two were nights that I really suffered. I noticed that there was an optimum time when I felt sleepy, and if I passed that because I wanted to watch "just another episode" of the latest box set, it would disrupt my body clock and I would be wide awake for a couple of hours more, even if I didn't want to be. I also noticed that particular activities—for example, becoming engrossed in drawing—would make me hyper-alert and energized, and that would affect my ability to fall asleep. These are just some examples of what I noticed about my habits. I stopped drinking red wine and also took steps to help with the menopause symptoms, benefiting my sleep quality. Of course, sometimes I do still stay up past my "bedtime," but I appreciate that there will be likely consequences, and so it becomes a conscious choice.

I do still suffer from insomnia from time to time, but I've got to know it better. I know that it's helpful to do certain things and avoid others as a way of increasing my chances of a good night's sleep. If I have trouble falling asleep or if I wake up, I avoid fighting it and instead see it as an opportunity to practice my mindfulness meditations.

I hope this book will awaken a sense of curiosity about your own relationship to sleep, and encourage you to explore another way of being awake … and asleep.

Anna Black

# HOW TO MAKE THE MOST OF THIS BOOK

This book is not going to fix your sleeping problems, but it will help you understand and manage them. You may have had trouble sleeping for quite a while, or it may be something new for you. Reading this book will not make your insomnia disappear by itself, but you will discover how practicing mindfulness meditation helps to reduce overall stress and changes our perception of difficulties in our life, as well as activating the body's internal calming response in times of stress. When we feel better able to handle the ups and downs of life, our sleep is more likely to improve.

Sleep is complex; many factors influence it, both within and out of our control, and you can learn more about this in Chapter 1. Then, in Chapter 2, you can gain an understanding of mindfulness, and why trying to meditate to go to sleep is not particularly helpful, because it introduces an attitude of striving for a particular outcome—in this case, falling asleep. We can't force ourselves to go to sleep—sleep comes over us without us making any effort. Rather than drawing on a bag of techniques to help us "in the moment," it is more helpful to explore a different way of being throughout our life—awake as well as asleep. Dr. Jason Ong, the developer of MBTI (Mindfulness-based Therapy for Insomnia; see page 55), says that insomnia is a 24-hour condition owing to the far-reaching impact it has on us. It therefore makes sense that our way of approaching it should be a 24-hour one, and cultivating mindfulness meditation is one way to do exactly that. The practices in Chapter 3 are designed to help you do this—you can bring them into everyday life as well as drawing upon them at times when you cannot sleep.

Chapter 4 teaches you how to create a sleep diary to observe what is actually happening when you have trouble sleeping. It encourages an attitude of curiosity, which is a key feature of mindfulness meditation.

## Getting help

Whether trouble sleeping is something new or a chronic problem, your first step should be to see your physician. As well as making sure that there is no underlying medical problem, he or she may prescribe sleeping tablets. These can be helpful, but it is important to be aware that they are highly addictive and so they should always be a short-term solution only.

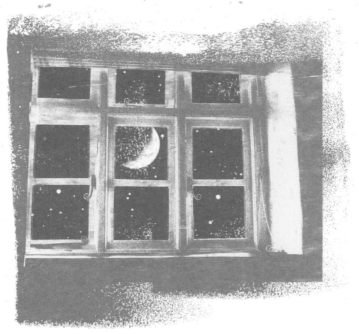

# CHAPTER 1
# ALL ABOUT SLEEP

This chapter gives you some background on why sleep is so important for physiological as well as performance reasons, and how sleep deprivation can seriously affect our mental and physical health and well-being. I encourage you to read this lightly. Adding worries about the effects of sleep deprivation to your repertoire is not helpful and potentially counterproductive.

The aim of this chapter is to demonstrate why we should prioritize sleep, to understand more about the body's amazing capacity to self-regulate and find its own rhythms, and to learn new ways that we can support rather than sabotage that.

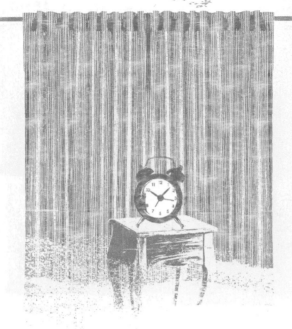

# THE IMPORTANCE OF SLEEP

**We spend about a quarter to a third of our lives asleep, but just because we are not awake doesn't mean that time is unproductive. The physiological changes that occur when we are asleep determine how well we feel and perform when we are awake.**

It's often said that diet, exercise, and sleep are the three foundational pillars to good health and well-being. While many of us understand the importance of eating a healthy, balanced diet and of keeping fit, we are perhaps less familiar with how important sleep is.

We've all experienced the effects of too little sleep: what it means for our mood, focus, and concentration, and also how it affects us physically—we have less energy, and feel tired and groggy. However, the importance of sleep and the consequences of being sleep-deprived go beyond this.

Sleep influences all the major systems in our body, and those systems in turn influence our sleep. Insufficient sleep can disrupt bodily functions that affect how we think and behave, and how we think and behave can disrupt our sleep. Therefore problems with sleeping can quickly become a vicious cycle.

At its simplest, sleep plays an important role in:

- Creating a healthy immune system
- Repairing muscle
- Consolidating learning and memory
- Regulating growth and appetite through the release of certain hormones
- Regulating mood and emotion.

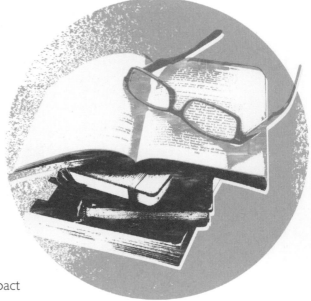

Sufficient sleep is essential to our well-being, both physically and emotionally, so it is not surprising that when we are deprived of it we feel the impact in all areas of our life. There is plenty of evidence

## The size of the problem

In a survey carried out in the USA in 2005, 75 percent of adults surveyed reported experiencing at least one symptom of a sleep problem a few nights a week in the previous month (National Sleep Federation, "Sleep America Poll," 2005). In the UK it is believed that 1 in 3 people experience problems sleeping, and the elderly are particularly affected.

that poor-quality or too little sleep can have serious consequences for our physical and mental health (see page 27).

Research on sleep usually measures objective and/or subjective sleep quality, and there is an important distinction between the two:

OBJECTIVE SLEEP QUALITY is assessed in laboratory conditions to determine the duration, efficiency, minimal broken sleep, and proper cycling through the different stages of n-REM and REM sleep (see pages 14–17).

SUBJECTIVE SLEEP QUALITY is our perception of how easily we fall asleep and whether it feels as if we had enough to feel rested throughout the day.

Problems with either can be debilitating, but the difference is significant in that, while it may be difficult to significantly improve sleep objectively for physiological reasons, we can change our perception of our sleep and its quality, and thereby our relationship with it. If we don't feel depleted by our experience, we are much more likely to view it neutrally or even favorably. This is where practicing mindfulness meditation may be particularly helpful, since with mindfulness we never "tackle" a problem in order to fix it. Instead, as we learn to accept it, our perception of the difficulty changes and it becomes less of a problem for us. However, we must practice mindfulness meditation to allow this to happen—we can't just tell ourselves to accept something. Acceptance arises from a raft of things coming together.

# WHAT HAPPENS WHEN WE SLEEP?

Until the early 20th century, when we became able to measure brain activity with electroencephalogram (EEG) rays, it was believed that during sleep the brain shut down and rested from the activity of the day. However, the reality is very different, and in fact the brain can be more active when we are asleep than when we are awake.

Whether we are awake or asleep depends on activity in specific areas of the brain. The part of the brain that promotes wakefulness also inhibits the part that promotes sleep activity, and vice versa. The shift between the different areas is caused by internal factors such as the circadian rhythm (see page 18) and the release of hormones, and is usually self-regulating. The drive to sleep increases the longer we are awake, and as we sleep it abates so that it is near zero when we wake.

Sleep, or more officially the Sleep Cycle, is made up of different stages of REM (rapid eye movement) and n-REM (non-rapid eye movement) sleep. Each cycle lasts about 90 minutes and is repeated three to six times each night. However, this cycle may be disrupted by stimulants such as coffee, nicotine, and alcohol, as well as by medical conditions and sleep deprivation.

We usually spend about 75 percent of the night in n-REM and 25 percent in REM sleep. Each of the different stages is as important as the others, and it is believed that the right balance of all the stages is crucial for restful and restorative sleep, which promotes learning, memory, and growth processes such as cell formation and repair, and regulates mood and the ability to concentrate.

The first cycle begins with a period of n-REM.

## N-REM

Characterized by a reduction in physiological activity in the body, sleep gradually becomes deeper and the brain waves slow, along with the breath, heart rate, and blood pressure. Although the following are listed as separate stages, they actually merge into one another.

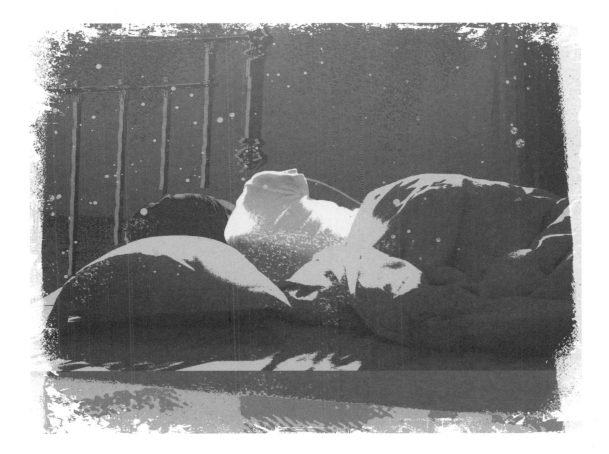

**N1 (STAGE 1)** Typically lasts 1–7 minutes, when we are hovering between being awake and falling asleep. If we are asleep, it is very light. We may experience sudden muscle jerks preceded by a falling sensation.

**N2 (STAGE 2)** Lasts about 10–25 minutes and signifies the onset of sleep. Eye movement stops, breath and heart rate become more regular, and body temperature drops. We have disengaged from our surroundings. Brain waves become slower, with occasional bursts of rapid activity. Spontaneous periods of muscle tension are interspersed with periods of muscle relaxation.

N3 (STAGE 3) Typically lasts 20–40 minutes and is also called "Slow Wave Sleep" (SWS). This is our deepest and most restorative sleep, and is believed to be associated with bodily recovery, certain types of learning, and changes to the central nervous system. Children experience the greatest amount of N3 sleep, which decreases with age. The longer someone has been awake, the more N3 sleep they get once N3 sleep occurs. It is harder to wake someone in this stage than in any other, since the brain is less responsive to external stimuli. If we are wakened in this stage, we may feel groggy and disoriented for a while.

Breathing becomes much slower, blood pressure drops, and muscles relax. There is decreased muscle activity, but they can still function. Blood supply to muscles increases. Hormones are released, including the growth hormone essential for muscle development. During this period tissue growth and repair occurs, and depleted energy is restored.

The majority of N3 sleep occurs in the first third of the night. N3 sleep typically takes up less time in the second cycle, and often disappears altogether in later cycles.

Then there is often a series of body movements that signal the ascent toward REM, moving through lighter n-REM. Often you "cycle back up" to N2 for 5–10 minutes before moving into the REM state.

## REM

REM sleep usually occurs about 90 minutes after falling asleep. It recurs every 90 minutes or so, and lasts longer as the night progresses. There is intense brain activity similar to when we are awake. This is when we are most likely to dream.

### Did you know?

Sleeping in a cooler room is helpful in facilitating the natural drop in body temperature that will encourage the onset of sleep.

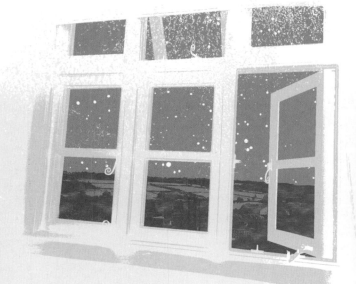

During REM sleep, breathing is faster, shallower, and more irregular. The heart rate and blood pressure increase, and the eyes often dart back and forth, causing the eyelids to flicker. Body temperature drops to its lowest point. Although the brain is awake, the body is paralyzed—a safety measure preventing us from acting out our dreams and perhaps causing injury.

It is thought that memories and learning are consolidated during REM sleep, that the body's brain chemistry is restored to a natural balance, and that mood is regulated (see page 27).

## RELEASE OF HORMONES

Hormones play an important role in regulating our sleepiness or wakefulness. During the various stages of sleep, some hormones are secreted and/or released and others are inhibited or reduced. These often determine how the body functions, for example suppressing appetite. When our sleep is disrupted, therefore, the hormones are unable to function as they should, and that can have a negative impact on our health and well-being. For instance, diabetes is caused by the body's inability to produce insulin, and insufficient sleep increases the risk of diabetes. However, those who sleep longer than 9 hours also seem to be at a greater risk of diabetes, so, where insulin is concerned, it seems to be the right balance of sleep that may be significant.

# HOW SLEEP IS REGULATED

The body has a built-in system called the circadian rhythm, which is responsible for regulating sleepiness and wakefulness over a 24-hour period (the time it takes for the Earth to circle the sun). The circadian rhythm usually emerges between two and six months after birth, and is controlled by the area of the brain that responds to light and receives input direct from the retina in the eye. It causes wakefulness to fluctuate through the day, and then, as darkness falls, it encourages sleepiness.

If we go to bed and rise at a regular time, we will help ourselves create and maintain a balanced circadian rhythm. It is easily disrupted by changes in sleeping or waking patterns, perhaps caused by shift work, late nights at weekends, traveling across time zones, stress, or illness. We can strengthen our circadian rhythm by following good sleeping habits (see page 36).

Our circadian rhythm can change over time. When we are younger we are more likely to be "night owls," staying up and rising later, and as we get older we are more likely to go to bed and rise earlier.

The circadian rhythm plays a role in some important systems that influence our sleeping habits, such as how much melatonin (see opposite) the body produces. It also regulates our core body temperature, so that it increases during the day and drops at night as we fall asleep. This then plays a role in helping us to stay asleep (hence the importance of maintaining a cool room). Our temperature usually begins to rise again at about 4am as we start to move from sleep to waking.

## Did you know?

To avoid an elevated body temperature at bedtime, if you are exercising, do so at least 4 hours before going to bed. Likewise, the best time for taking a hot bath is about 60–90 minutes before bedtime. It is not the raised body temperature from the bath that makes us sleepy, but the subsequent drop as we cool down.

## MELATONIN

Melatonin is a hormone that helps to regulate our sleep/wake cycle. Its production is influenced by the circadian rhythm and the amount of light we are exposed to. Melatonin is released in the dark and suppressed by light. Therefore the level is at its lowest first thing in the morning, and rises toward evening as darkness falls. It remains elevated through the night—helping us to sleep—but then falls in the early morning.

The long, dark nights and shorter days of winter affect the production of melatonin, and that can result in changes to our mood and energy levels (known as seasonal affective disorder or SAD). Melatonin is also degraded by stress, which is a common trigger for sleep problems.

Melatonin can also be taken as a pill, and is available over the counter in the USA and elsewhere. However, in the UK it is available exclusively by prescription as a short-term sleeping aid only, and is not recommended for those under the age of 55.

# WHAT STOPS US FROM SLEEPING?

**Many factors affect our ability to sleep. Some are beyond our control, and it becomes a question of learning how to live with their consequences, but others are related to lifestyle, so we can do something about them.**

## AGE

As we get older, our total sleep time and the period we spend in deep Slow Wave Sleep (see page 16) decreases. Since we are less likely to be woken by external stimuli when we are in deep sleep, the number of times we wake up increases and sleep becomes fragmented. Once we are awake it also takes us longer to fall back to sleep. This may all be caused by lifestyle changes, such as retirement, as well as increased health problems and the side effects of medication, but many people find that they need less sleep as they become older, too. Women may experience night sweats and poorer sleep overall with the onset of the menopause.

## MEDICAL DISORDERS

Those that affect sleep include apnea (when a person's airway becomes blocked or obstructed, resulting in shallow breathing or even a temporary stop in breathing, which disrupts sleep), mental-health disorders such as depression and anxiety, obesity, and pain.

## WORK

Shift work can be particularly disruptive, but working long or irregular hours can adversely affect the body's natural rhythms.

## ENVIRONMENT

This might be a room that is too warm, external noise (airplanes, neighbors, traffic), or perhaps a snoring partner or one who also has difficulty sleeping.

## TRAVEL

Crossing time zones disrupts our internal body clock, which regulates sleep and waking.

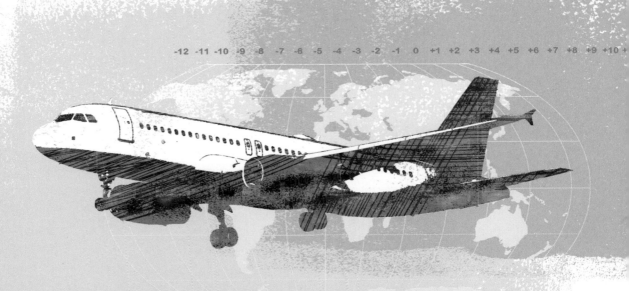

-12 -11 -10 -9 -8 -7 -6 -5 -4 -3 -2 -1 0 +1 +2 +3 +4 +5 +6 +7 +8 +9 +10+

180° 165° 150° 135° 120° 105° 90° 75° 60° 45° 30° 15° 0° 15° 30° 45° 60° 75° 90° 105° 120° 135° 150° 165° 180°
24   1    2    3    4    5    6   7   8   9   10  11  12  13  14  15  16  17  18  19   20   21   22   23   24

## STRESS

This could be caused by relationship problems, work (or lack of work after retirement), bereavement, and young children, among other factors. Worrying can keep us awake and stress degrades melatonin, which is essential for sleep (see page 19).

## INSOMNIA

This condition is when you have trouble falling asleep or staying asleep, when you wake very early, and/or when you don't feel satisfied with the quality of your sleep. If this persists for a month or more, it becomes a chronic condition. People experiencing insomnia often feel that their mind is racing, and get caught up in spirals of worry and negative thinking. This state of arousal keeps them awake.

What we experience may vary according to age. Adolescents are more likely to have problems falling asleep; having trouble staying asleep, or waking very early, is more common in older people.

Although we may think of insomnia as being a nighttime problem, it's actually a 24-hour condition. When we don't sleep well at night, in the daytime we tend to experience fatigue, lack of energy, sleepiness, decrease in concentration and/or memory, and disturbances in mood and motivation (see page 27).

Insomnia is one of the earliest and most common symptoms of stress, and it is also associated with pre-existing conditions such as anxiety, depression, and pain. In addition, if you suffer from these conditions you are more at risk of insomnia. Because of the way sleep, pain, and psychological distress are interlinked, combined approaches to treatment are more successful and therefore recommended.

That is one reason why mindfulness-based approaches may be particularly helpful (see pages 53–55).

THE COST OF INSOMNIA In the UK, 1 in 3 adults reports problems sleeping. Insomnia is the most common sleep complaint in the USA and affects as many as 30 million people (just over 1 in 10 adults). The cost in terms of the productivity of the American workforce is estimated to be around $63.2 billion, and consumers spend another $32 billion on sleep-aid products. However, many of us don't realize that there are very practical things we can do to improve our sleep by simply exploring different habits and behavior (see page 36), rather than spending money on sleep-aid products. Research shows that regularly restricting our sleep by an hour has a negative impact on our attention, reaction times, mood, and sleepiness, so allowing just one hour more for sleep can make a difference to how we feel, as well as have long-term benefits.

## LIFESTYLE

Partying late, watching the latest box set, or spending long hours at a computer, plus drinking alcohol or caffeine or taking other stimulants are all factors that can affect sleep. Plus, when we have trouble sleeping, we may inadvertently employ strategies that make it worse, thereby fueling rather than reducing our sleep debt.

ALCOHOL Many of us enjoy a drink or two as a way of winding down at the end of a long and stressful day, or perhaps to self-medicate against chronic aches and pains. However, although alcohol might help us to get to sleep initially, an alcohol-induced sleep will be lighter and more fragmented. This blocks the early, most restorative stages of sleep and inhibits the release of growth hormones that occur during the night.

As alcohol levels in the blood drop, we are more likely to experience periods of wakefulness. In addition, alcohol is a diuretic, so it will also disrupt our sleep by increasing the need to urinate during the night. If you or your partner snore or suffer from sleep apnea (see page 20), this condition may be exacerbated by alcohol.

CAFFEINE Coffee is often the go-to drink to kick-start the morning, and there is no doubt that it can help to wake us up. It stays in the body for 12 hours, however, so drinking coffee or other caffeinated drinks during the day or in the evening inhibits and disrupts the body's self-regulating wake/sleep systems for longer than you might think.

Caffeine can also be found in chocolate, black tea, energy drinks, and many sodas. The last is particularly significant for children and teenagers, and so should be reduced in the evening as part of a good sleep hygiene routine (see page 37).

How caffeine affects us may change as we get older. I used to be able to drink coffee after an evening meal, but now late afternoon is my cut-off point. It is worth reviewing your habits and behavior periodically so that you can respond to your changing requirements.

## Try this

Pay attention to what you are drinking in an evening and how much, and notice whether it affects your sleep. You may notice that certain drinks affect you more or less. Approach it as an experiment and be as objective as possible. You can use a Sleep Diary to keep track of this (see Chapter 4).

# THE EFFECT OF TECHNOLOGY

**For most of us, the days when bedrooms were simply places to sleep and make love are long gone. First it was the appearance of the television, then the smartphone, laptop, e-reader, and tablet. All are now commonplace in our bedrooms.**

There is nothing wrong with the technology or the objects themselves. It's simply that the presence of these items immediately signals activity—doing something—rather than resting or letting go of activity. Also, the way we engage with them can have a negative impact on our sleep.

A smartphone, laptop, tablet, or television screen acts as a mini sun, emitting blue light that interferes with the production of melatonin that is essential for becoming sleepy (see page 19). While on some phones it is possible to activate a nighttime filter that reduces the blue light, it doesn't remove it entirely.

The gadgets themselves are a source of distraction. Checking emails and status updates on social media keeps us in a state of hyperarousal. The brain remains on alert for what might pop into our inbox or social media feed, rather than being encouraged to wind down in preparation for sleep.

Using a smartphone for work keeps us connected mentally long after we have physically left the office. It becomes harder to disconnect from work during the evening, and that can lead to rumination that disrupts sleep. If you work from home, it is even more important to give yourself a mental break by making a clear distinction between work and leisure hours.

Notifications and alerts can interrupt our sleep. Healthy sleepers will experience up to ten brief arousals or awakenings per hour of sleep. These usually last only seconds, and they are often associated with body movement. Their fleeting nature means they are usually forgotten, and so we are unaware of them unless they are prolonged because of a sound or other factor such as smell. If an alert sounds on your phone during one of these mini awakenings, you are more likely to wake up properly. If you are someone who experiences problems with sleeping, this can set off the reactive pattern of insomnia (see page 21).

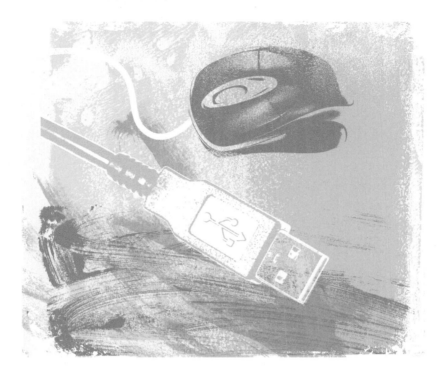

## TECHNOLOGY AND CHILDREN

Today's young people, from toddlers to teens, are the first generation to have used technology from an early age, and in an era when both parents often work. This can result in parenting being squeezed into fewer hours, and technology being used for childcare as an essential part of this juggling act.

It is not just watching television before bedtime that affects the child's sleep. Simply being in the same room as a television that is on will have a similar effect. If a child has trouble sleeping, this will affect the parents' sleep, too.

More than 80 percent of children in the UK have a cellphone by the age of 12, and this rises to 90 percent by the age of 15 (Censuswide Research, 2016). Most children use their phones beyond bedtime, with the same consequences as adults, although for children it will be the interaction with their peers via social media that may fuel rumination and anxiety, rather than the problems of the workplace.

### Did you know?

Hospital attendance for children with sleep problems has tripled in the UK in the last ten years, and across the world children are sleeping less than previous generations.

## Don't take someone else's word for it

One of the over-arching principles of mindfulness meditation is to explore your own experience. It is always useful for us to bring our own habits of using technology into awareness and notice how they affect us. We then have a choice about what to do with this feedback. There is a practice for doing this (see page 100).

As role models, this is a great opportunity for parents to set an example, and the experiment can also be done as a family. Each person, whatever their age, will notice the night- and daytime effects of cutting back on technology in the hours before bedtime.

Young people are more likely to have problems falling asleep than to wake up once they are asleep. Research suggests that sleeping one hour less over three consecutive nights significantly affects their performance in terms of memory, focus, attention, and problem-solving. This isn't surprising: During puberty and adolescence, the brain goes through major change, restructuring and rewiring itself, and long, deep sleep is essential for rest and recovery.

It is believed that one of the functions of sleep is to consolidate daytime learning and memories and hardwire them into long-term memory so they can be retrieved when necessary. If sleep is disrupted, learning cannot be processed in the same way. In addition, tiredness leads to a drop in energy during the day, and that affects attention and focus and makes learning more difficult.

If sleep is repeatedly shortened or disrupted by the use of technology, there is an increased risk of associated health problems, particularly obesity (see page 30). However, it is relatively easy to start prioritizing and instigating healthier habits around the use of technology and a child's nighttime routine.

# WHAT HAPPENS WHEN WE DON'T GET ENOUGH SLEEP?

Many people don't realize that sleep is one of the cornerstones of well-being, along with diet and exercise. We may be aware that regularly eating junk food and not exercising affects our physical and mental well-being, but we may not make the same connection with not getting enough sleep. Although this is an emerging field in research, with new discoveries being made all the time, it is known that sleep is closely linked to all the body's physiological systems, and so when sleep is disrupted, it is inevitable that we don't function at our best, emotionally, mentally, and physically.

## EMOTIONS AND MOOD

We have all experienced how we become more irritable and reactive when we are lacking sleep and there is usually a decline in mood as well. We are more likely to rate our mood negatively after one night of sleep deprivation. Laboratory studies suggest that when we are deprived of sleep we may become more intolerant of and frustrated with others, more likely to blame others for hypothetical predicaments, and less likely to compromise in order to find a mutually satisfying outcome. We also lack empathy and are more self-centered.

## THE BRAIN AND PERFORMANCE

Lack of sleep particularly affects basic attention and vigilance, the cornerstones for more complex thinking. The ability to maintain sustained attention is also critical in many industries where work involves monitoring, so poor sleep can have an impact on safety as well as performance.

Most of us begin to experience slower reactions and responses after we have been awake for 16 hours, and this increases as wakefulness persists. Even restricting sleep by a couple of hours in a night can lead to significant lengthening of reaction times. If we sleep six hours a night for two weeks, our performance will be impaired to the same degree as if we had been awake for 48 hours non-stop.

It also seems that slower response times are associated with greater activation of the default mode regions of the brain. This may suggest that as we become more tired the brain is unable to allocate tasks to its most appropriate and effective processing areas. Rather than making the most of our brain's resources, we default to the most basic processing, which requires less energy and effort.

Although the pre-frontal cortex appears to be particularly affected by sleep deprivation, the evidence does not show clearly how the brain's executive functions are affected. It seems that some types of thinking are affected more than others by sleep deprivation: More creative, flexible, and innovative aspects are degraded particularly, as well as those that rely on emotional data.

The pre-frontal cortex plays a role in emotional processing, inhibiting connections with the more primitive areas of the brain like the amygdala (which activates the stress reaction cycle; see page 46). If these connections are impaired, effective emotional processing will be too. The more we get caught up in negative thinking, the narrower our perspective on the world becomes. Mindfulness can play a part in remedying that (see page 53).

Our ability to learn new things and remember them is essential for basic survival as well as performance. Sleep is crucial in preparing the brain to acquire new information *before* learning, and it also plays an essential role *afterward*, consolidating learning and integrating it into long-term memory banks, from where it can be retrieved when it is needed. If these two stages are disrupted by sleep deprivation, the development of new memories—and therefore learning—will be hindered. Next time you are studying for an exam, starting a new job, or learning a new skill, invest in your sleep before and after to help you get the most out of it.

The emotional content of the memories is also affected by sleep deprivation. It appears that positive and neutral memories are more susceptible than negative memories, so if we are deprived of sleep our positive and neutral memories are more likely to be degraded and lost. That leaves us with a preponderance of negative memories. As human beings, we already have a natural negativity bias in our thinking, which is tied into our essential survival wiring—it is more important to remember where a potential threat is located than the experience of watching a beautiful sunrise. People who practice mindfulness often comment on how they begin to notice the small positive experiences that occur throughout the day, but that are commonly missed in the busy-ness of life. This helps counteract the natural negativity bias. Once we consciously notice a happy experience, it becomes banked into our long-term memory.

## Sleep affects thinking and performance

An interesting study by Harrison & Horne (1999) exploring the effect of sleep loss on performance involved ten participants playing a "dynamic and realistic marketing decision-making 'game'" that required flexible thinking and updating of plans in the light of new information. Compared to the way they performed when well rested, when sleep-deprived the participants showed significantly greater rigidity of thought, remained stuck on unsuccessful strategies that were no longer effective, were inefficient at updating plans to take account of new information, and failed to develop innovative solutions. In fact, their performance declined to the extent that they became "financially insolvent" after 32–36 hours of being awake, whereas the same participants performed well—and even made a profit—when well rested.

Clearly there are significant limitations with the study in terms of generalizing conclusions, but it is an interesting example of how sleep deprivation may affect individuals in real scenarios.

## OBESITY

People who haven't had enough sleep have reduced levels of the hormone leptin, which is responsible for suppressing appetite, and an increase in the peptide ghrelin, which stimulates it. Therefore chronic sleep deprivation may cause us to eat more and gain weight. It may also cause us to make unhealthy food choices. In addition, if we are overweight we are more likely to have problems sleeping.

Sleep apnea (see page 20) can increase the risk of obesity. The excessive sleepiness caused by apnea inhibits the desire to exercise, which contributes to being overweight.

## IMMUNE SYSTEM AND PAIN

"Sleep is the best medicine" is not an old wives' tale. The proper functioning of the body's immune system is compromised by poor sleep. Both total sleep time and Slow Wave Sleep (see page 16) are essential when battling acute infection, and both are disrupted by pain and illness, which can delay healing.

There is an association between lack of sleep and an increase in spontaneous pain, as well as general physical discomfort, headaches, and muscle and stomach pain.

## A SUMMARY

We have learnt that when we are sleep deprived:

- We become more easily distracted, and for longer periods
- The brain is not primed for learning and is unable to consolidate effectively what is learned, thereby affecting long-term memory
- We experience an increasingly negative bias in mood and memory
- Our appetite increases, so we eat more and make unhealthier choices
- Our energy levels drop and so we exercise less
- We experience pain more acutely
- Our immune system is compromised
- Essential hormones go out of kilter, which can affect growth, reproduction, and other bodily functions, along with the metabolism of glucose, which can lead to diabetes.

These negative effects often remain even when alertness and vigilance are restored with stimulants such as caffeine. Therefore, although we may feel more awake and alert, behind the scenes the body's systems are not functioning at their best or even properly.

## Try this

As you are reading this section, what are you noticing about your response to it? First take a moment to become aware of the story that is playing out in your head, noticing any emotions arising or felt sensations in the body. Notice if you are catastrophizing about what you are reading and thinking of the long-term consequences of not getting enough sleep; or perhaps you feel a sense of recognition or familiarity—ah, that's why I do that! It can be reassuring to know that our behavior is a consequence of the body's systems being out of kilter. As always, bring a sense of friendly interest to this reflection.

Now reflect on how your mood and emotions are usually affected by not getting enough sleep. How about your performance and the way you interact with others? Are you more reactive and less compassionate toward others? If you are not sure, then just start doing this type of reflection at different times—when you are fresh and awake as well as tired and sleepy—and notice how your performance, mood, and relationships with others may be affected.

Remember that there is no need to be critical about what you discover, but instead bring an attitude of curiosity and self-compassion to the experiment and simply acknowledge how things are. This is about becoming familiar with our habitual patterns and bringing them into awareness. Doing this can help us spot them earlier so they become useful "red flags," warning us that perhaps things are out of kilter and we need to take some wise action.

Practicing mindfulness should not be seen as a means of getting by with less sleep, but rather about waking up so that we are more likely to notice how our behavior and performance changes when we are sleep deprived—and can then do something about it. That might mean not putting ourselves or others at risk by doing certain tasks such as driving when sleepy or simply acknowledging that when we are over-tired we will be more reactive and less tolerant of others, as well as doing what we can to address our lack of sleep.

# HOW MUCH SLEEP DO WE NEED?

There is no "golden" number of hours that is the perfect amount of sleep, and subjective sleep quality (whether we feel we have had a good night's sleep or not) is as significant as duration. Two people can sleep for a similar amount of time with similar periods of wakefulness, and yet perceive it very differently.

In general, eight hours is usually quoted for adults; children and young adults will need more and the elderly less. However, it is important not to get too hooked on numbers, particularly if you do have trouble sleeping, since there may be a tendency to constantly measure how you are doing and then feel disappointed if you are falling short. This may create additional anxiety about sleeping, and that is unhelpful. Mindfulness helps us to let go of particular expectations and of striving toward a particular goal, and instead helps us to be okay with the way things actually are.

Ask yourself the following questions after an average night's sleep:
- Do I feel healthy and happy?
- Do I depend on caffeine to get through the day (particularly first thing in the morning)?

## Did you know?

The notion of sleeping through the night for a particular number of hours is a relatively modern one. Historically, humans slept in two bouts. The first sleep began soon after dusk. There would then be a waking period when people would have sex, or perhaps even get up, go out and socialize, before retiring for a second sleep in the early hours before dawn. Modern-day sleeping patterns have emerged only since the Industrial Revolution enabled everyone, not just the very rich, to manipulate light and therefore extend the "day."

- Do I feel sleepy during the day? (This is usually a sign that you are not getting enough sleep.)

Depending on your answers, you may decide to make sleep a priority in your life.

## YOUR IDEAL AMOUNT OF SLEEP

Try this to work out the number of hours' sleep that is best for you:

**STEP 1** Pay off any sleep debt by getting plenty of sleep. You may need to do this while you're on vacation!

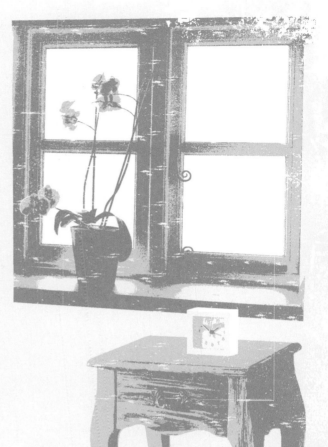

**STEP 2** Using 7½ hours as a starting point, count back from the time you need to get up and make that your bedtime (factor in a short period of "falling-asleep time").

**STEP 3** Begin going to bed at that time for at least a week or, better still, ten days, and notice whether you begin waking up just before your alarm.

If after ten days you still need the alarm, go to bed a little earlier and continue until you find the right duration for you.

If you have the flexibility to get up at any time, another option is to go to bed at the same time each night and notice when you wake up naturally, without any outside interference. Doing this over a period of a couple weeks will allow you to determine how much sleep you personally need.

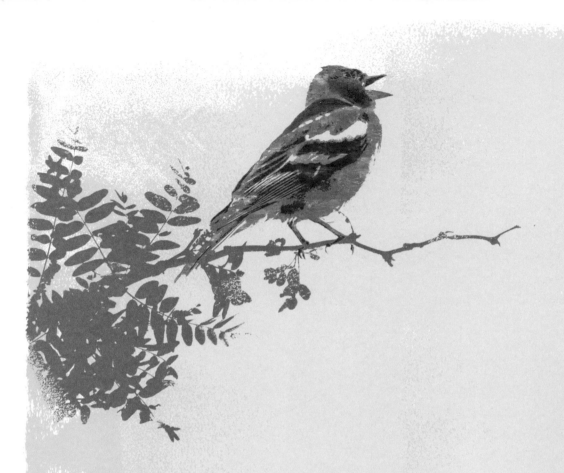

The test is sleeping for a particular length of time and waking naturally (without an alarm) feeling refreshed, without needing any stimulants such as caffeine. However, you may want to have an alarm clock set as a back-up!

For some people, it's not just the duration that matters but the timing. Night owls and early birds may have to change the time they go to bed in order to accommodate that, and that will affect when they rise (assuming they still want to achieve their particular ideal duration). As always, have some fun experimenting with what works for you.

## WHY ARE SOME OF US "NIGHT OWLS" AND OTHERS "EARLY BIRDS"?

We have already seen that our internal body clock, or circadian rhythm, is set to approximately 24 hours. However, if your clock runs faster than that you are more likely to be an early bird and wake up early. Night owls' clocks run more slowly, and they prefer going to bed later. Although we may have a genetic predisposition to be one or the other, we still can exert some control. For example, if you are a night owl who has to get up early for work, employing good sleep hygiene habits (see page 36) will help to override your natural tendency to stay up late, ensuring that you are not short-changed on your sleep.

## IS NAPPING HELPFUL?

Be aware that if you suffer from insomnia, napping may make it more difficult for you to fall asleep at night, and may thereby exacerbate the situation.

In many cultures, an afternoon siesta is built into everyday rhythms, often as a practical response to a hot climate. Many people report feeling more alert and rested after a nap, and it can be a good way to pay back some of your sleep debt, but the key is to keep it short, ideally no more than 20 minutes. Nap for much longer and you risk falling into deep sleep, which may leave you feeling groggy when you wake.

## CATCH-UP SLEEP

Many of us try to make the most of the weekend or days off by lying in to catch up on sleep. However, this may not be helpful, because it disrupts our body clock. As we get older, our ability to sleep in and catch up on sleep is much reduced. It is much better if you can stick to your usual time of getting up and going to bed, even at weekends.

### Did you know?

You can buy daylight alarm clocks that mimic the rising sun, gradually increasing to full strength at the alarm time. By using light to wake ourselves up, we are tapping into the body's own internal systems regulated by the circadian rhythm. Personally, I find this a much gentler and more restful way to wake up than a strident alarm call.

# GOOD SLEEP HYGIENE

**Although we can feel powerless in the face of poor sleep, there are some simple changes we can make to ensure that we are supporting rather than undermining our body's internal sleep systems.**

People commonly report that implementing good sleeping habits is helpful. However, if you find your sleep does not improve despite making and maintaining lifestyle changes, it is recommended that you consult your physician.

Make sleep a priority—remind yourself that it is as important as exercising and eating well.

## COOL DOWN

Body temperature plays an important role in sleep. We fall asleep as our body temperature drops, and a lower body temperature also helps us to stay asleep before it begins to rise in the early hours as we waken. You can encourage a drop in body temperature deliberately by taking a hot bath or shower about an hour before bedtime and then making sure your environment is cool (about 63°F/17°C). As the body cools, you will begin to feel sleepy. Ideally, exercise no less than 4 hours before going to bed, to avoid elevating your core temperature.

## ENVIRONMENT

Sleep in a cool, dark room that is free of technology and has a comfortable bed. Turn any clocks to the wall to avoid watching the minutes in the early hours.

## DON'T SPEND TOO LONG IN BED

If our mood is low, we may retreat to bed rather than face the world. However, going to bed too early means repeated awakenings and a much shallower sleep, and we thereby miss out on restorative Slow Wave Sleep (see page 16).

## KEEP TO A REGULAR SCHEDULE

Stabilize your circadian rhythm by going to bed and getting up at the same time—even at weekends and when on vacation.

## GO TO BED WHEN YOU ARE SLEEPY

Listen to your body, and go to bed when you are sleepy. Likewise, don't go to bed before you are sleepy.

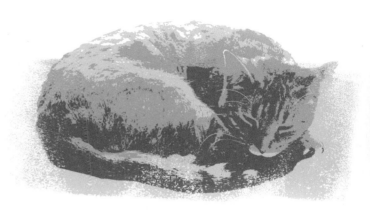

## AVOID STIMULANTS

Alcohol, caffeine, nicotine, and other stimulants are best avoided in the evening and perhaps even in the afternoon. Notice how you are affected. It is important to check ingredients—you may be surprised how prevalent caffeine is. It can be found in chocolate, many sodas, and even energy drinks.

## NOTICE WHAT YOU EAT

Certain types of food eaten too near bedtime can affect your sleep, but they can affect everyone differently, so if you think food may be a factor pay attention to what you eat when completing your Sleep Diary (see Chapter 4).

## AVOID TRYING TO SLEEP

Actively trying to fall asleep will only make you more awake, particularly because you may begin to feel anxious that you are not falling asleep. If you are awake, be awake. Read, get up, meditate, or do some yoga or other calming activity.

## REDUCE SCREEN TIME

Avoid screen time (including television and cellphones) an hour before bedtime, if possible.

## PROTECT YOUR WIND-DOWN TIME

Notice what helps you to move from the busy-ness of the day to winding down toward bedtime. Avoid or keep to a minimum activities that keep you buzzing. However, notice if there is a sense of striving when it comes to doing particular activities or behaving in a particular way, with the expectation that they will lead to a good night's sleep. This is unhelpful too.

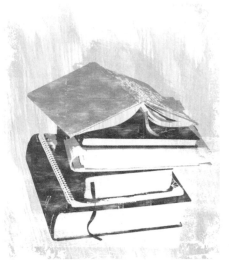

## CHAPTER 2
# INTRODUCING MINDFULNESS

Discover how mindfulness works and find out how developing a regular mindfulness practice during the day will benefit you overall, as well as giving you skills to draw on when you find yourself awake at night. Here you will find suggestions for particular ways to approach your mindfulness practice and helpful attitudes to cultivate.

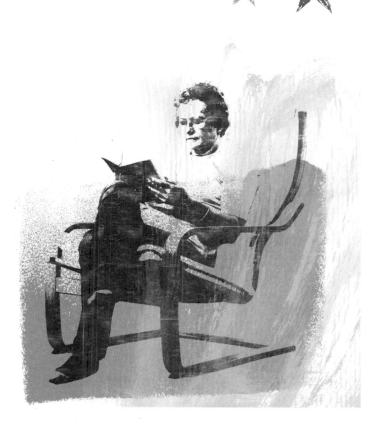

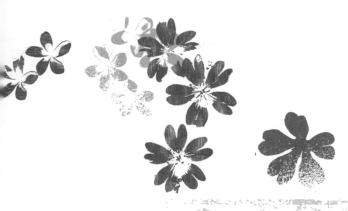

# WHAT IS MINDFULNESS?

**Mindfulness is intentionally paying attention to your experience
as it arises, without judging it.**

Most of the time what we experience just feels like a big blob. However, when we start paying attention we realize that our experience is multi-layered: It is made up of inner and outer experiences, and strands within them. Our inner experience consists of thoughts, emotions, and physical sensations; our outer experience is made up of the environment, behavior, and actions (our own and those of other people). All these arise individually and simultaneously, and interact with and influence one another.

How we pay attention is crucial. We want to notice whatever is arising without judging it, and actively cultivate attitudes of kindness and gentleness to what we notice. When we start practicing mindfulness, the first thing we often notice is how judgmental we are—judging situations, others, and, of course, ourselves. It is easy to fall into the trap of judging ourselves for being so judgmental! However, there is a difference between judging and discerning, and there is nothing wrong with having preferences.

We can cultivate the quality of mindfulness through practicing meditation, both formal (a regular practice that might include sitting practice, movement—yoga, walking, tai chi, qiqong—or a body scan) and informal, when we pay attention to what we are doing while we are doing it as we go about our day. Both types of practice are valuable and support each other.

## The origins of mindfulness

The recent popularity of mindfulness may lead you to think that it is something new, but it is quite the opposite. Mindfulness is a quality within us all, but it can be cultivated consciously through meditation, and this has been practiced for thousands of years. The secular form of mindfulness meditation that we discuss here came to the West more than 30 years ago and was developed by Dr. Jon Kabat-Zinn and his colleagues at the University of Massachusetts Hospital as a way of helping patients with chronic medical conditions learn to live with them. Since then its use has spread, and adapted mindfulness-based approaches are being used for medical disorders such as depression, anxiety, addiction, cancer, and pain, among many others, as well as in mainstream contexts such as schools, prisons, government, the workplace, and the sports arena. One reason that it has been accepted into such a diverse range of areas is the strong evidence for its efficacy. This is growing all the time, particularly in new areas, and mindfulness and sleep is one of those.

## THE BENEFITS OF FORMAL MEDITATION PRACTICE

When we practice formally, we are practicing focusing our attention on something in particular (such as the breath, physical sensations, sounds, or thoughts) for a certain amount of time. The regularity of the practice is more important than the duration, so try to do it a few times a week if you can't do it every day. It is better to sit for a shorter time, perhaps 5 minutes to begin with, and build it up, rather than struggle to sit for 30 minutes and feel that you have failed.

When we meditate, our mind will wander sooner rather than later, and at some point we notice that. This is a moment of pure awareness—we are in the present moment and we know that we are thinking. We acknowledge that we are "thinking" and bring our attention back to the focus, whatever that is. If we practice regularly, we end up doing this thousands of times. Every time we bring the attention back we are practicing letting go of a distraction, encouraging the unconscious mind to notice mind-wandering (which is why it is important not to beat ourselves up about it), practicing deliberately placing our attention where we want it to be, and cultivating attitudes of kindness, gentleness, curiosity, patience, letting go, acceptance, and non-striving. Therefore every time we exercise this muscle of awareness, we lay down new neural pathways in the brain: We change our brain and the way it works, and the evidence supports this (see pages 52–53).

Much of our day-to-day stress is caused by trying to control our experience, and particularly by things not being as we would like them to be, and the same thing happens at night if we are not sleeping as we think we should. When we meditate regularly, we notice how our experience is always changing. We become more comfortable with change and realize that we can't control our experience. When we struggle with not sleeping, we can get into a vicious cycle of trying to control all the elements that may influence sleep; but actually, this undermines it.

As we meditate, every state of mind will arise at some point: physical discomfort, boredom, restlessness, irritation, calm, peace, ease … Learning to explore these different states "on the mat" in a safe environment gives us the opportunity to practice being with them. Through noticing how they manifest in the body and how we habitually react to them, and through meeting them, we learn a different way to respond to them. Thus, when the same states of mind arise in everyday life, we are already familiar with them.

There is also an important element of showing up to practice. If we establish a regular meditation practice (maybe just 10–15 minutes a day), we do it regardless of whether we are in the mood. This is important: It cultivates a willingness to be with whatever shows up, however we are, and it can be helpful when we experience a bout of insomnia or face unexpected events.

## Reacting vs responding

When we react to something, it is automatic and unconscious. We usually don't have any control, since the reaction happens instantly, without awareness. However, a response is more considered. It arises from a pause or space that creates a moment of awareness about what is unfolding, and this allows us to make a choice about how we want to respond. This pause arises from regular meditation.

We often find it easier to pay attention to our experience if we make a specific time to do so, without any distractions, and setting aside a time to meditate allows this. Many people find it harder to practice mindfulness informally, because they get caught up in the busy-ness of the day and simply forget. That is not to say that if you meditate regularly but never practice informally you won't experience the benefits—you will, but you will gain even more if you can do both.

## THE BENEFITS OF INFORMAL PRACTICE

Sometimes we can have a strong formal meditation practice and yet, once we leave the house, we forget everything we've learned. "I'm too busy to be present at work or looking after the kids," we tell ourselves. It is challenging, but these are the times when we need mindfulness most and when it can be most beneficial.

If we can become used to practicing mindfulness throughout our day, it will become integrated into our lives. We will notice the benefits of pausing occasionally and acknowledging where we are and how best to respond, rather than reacting automatically and unconsciously. We find that we become aware of the fleeting positive moments that punctuate our day and that are often lost to us because we don't notice them.

The instruction for practicing informally is simple: Know what you are doing while you are doing it. If you are eating, for example, savor that mouthful, exploring taste, smell, texture, and sound, while paying attention to what is arising in your head, heart, and body in response. It is not about making yourself *like* the experience. You may not, and that's okay. It's simply about being *aware* of your experience as it arises.

The way you do it is important, too, and we consciously cultivate attitudes of kindness, non-striving, and letting go of the outcome. You can read more about these on pages 50–52. You can practice informally for just a minute or two, or for longer.

OUR MOOD AFFECTS OUR FRAME OF MIND Whether we practice formally or informally, mindfulness always allows us the opportunity to notice how our thoughts are influenced by our frame of mind. When we are in a good mood, we are better able to deal with challenges. When we are feeling tired, down, or stressed, we tend to see things negatively. We focus on and actively look for evidence that supports the negative story we are telling ourselves, and discount anything that contradicts it.

NOT A QUICK FIX It is important to acknowledge that mindfulness is not a quick fix. It takes time to begin undoing the habits of a lifetime, and it is important to be patient and let go of striving for a particular outcome. The pitfalls of practicing with a goal in mind are discussed on page 50.

THE IMPORTANCE OF PRACTICE Practicing regularly is crucial if we are to allow change to happen. We are setting ourselves up for disappointment if we think that all we need to do to fall asleep instantly is to tune into the breath. Paying attention is simple, but as human beings we throw in a lot of extra stuff that complicates it, and practicing regularly helps us to see that. It is also important to continue to practice even after things start to improve. Sleeping poorly is a 24-hour problem, and mindfulness has the potential to offer a 24-hour solution. All the research showing the benefits of mindfulness to those suffering from poor sleep includes regular meditation practice.

# HOW DOES MINDFULNESS HELP?

According to Mindful Nation UK, mindfulness training teaches people to become more aware of their thoughts, emotions, and body sensations, as well as being less reactive and judgmental toward them. They start recognizing thoughts as mental events rather than facts, and discover ways of dealing with automatic reactions to stress. They also become able to notice pleasant events and enjoy them, and develop a greater overall attitude of unconditional kindness, both toward themselves and others. The result of this is that they respond to their own experience, and to events in their lives and the people around them, in a healthier and more compassionate way.

Whatever brings us to mindfulness—anxiety, pain, sleeplessness, or something else—we never actually try to "fix" that particular problem. Instead, we learn to relate to our "suffering"—whether physical or psychological—in a different way. Forcing ourselves to fall asleep (or resisting being awake) is a non-starter. Learning how to move from a place of resisting or not wanting our experience to one of allowing it to be (since it's already here) is at the heart of mindfulness practice. Paradoxically, by letting go of the need to fall asleep you may find that your sleep improves. Regardless of this, however, acceptance involves letting go of the mental struggle that can be so exhausting, and therefore you may feel less tired even if you are not actually sleeping more.

# ACCEPTING THINGS AS THEY ARE

If we are awake when we should be asleep, things are definitely not as we would like them to be. This scenario can generate a range of emotions, including frustration, irritation, and anger, each feeding on the others, creating tension and discomfort in the body as well as an agitated mind. Being awake is most likely unavoidable—you are just awake—but how we respond to being awake is within our control. We can respond as described, with all the negativity and suffering that brings, or we can choose a different approach. We can acknowledge that we are awake and let go of striving to fall asleep or catastrophizing about it. Then, all we are left with is being awake. We know how to do this; perhaps we can meditate, read a book, do some yoga stretches—do something that you enjoy or something that you will feel good about doing. You may feel sleepy in due course, but you may not—and that's okay. We are not "doing" in order to fall asleep, but simply "being" awake. When we are tired, we accept that we are tired rather than railing against it and making ourselves feel bad about it.

# FIGHT OR FLIGHT: ACTIVATING THE CALMING RESPONSE

Insomnia is often triggered by a stressful event—perhaps worries about work, money, or family matters—or by illness or pain. The anxiety these thoughts generate activates the body's defense system (known as the Fight or Flight reaction). The stress reaction causes the body to release various stress hormones, including adrenaline and cortisol. Cortisol is one of the hormones that is released by the circadian rhythm, and contributes to

## Try this

Next time you find yourself catastrophizing about being awake when you'd rather be sleeping, notice how you are relating to being awake. What are you noticing in the head (thoughts), heart (emotions), and body (physical sensations). There is no need to judge what you find. Simply notice how uncomfortable resisting our experience can be.

wakefulness. Adrenaline ensures that we are hyper-alert and wired for action—the antithesis of sleepiness. Melatonin (see page 19), the hormone that increases in response to darkness and causes sleepiness, is degraded by stress. So feeling stressed causes us to be more alert and inhibits the body's natural sleep system; our potential for sleep is therefore being undermined from two sides. The negative daytime consequences of sleep disruption generate more anxiety as we worry about not sleeping again, activating the stress reaction once more, and therefore our fears are realized when we can't sleep. And so the cycle continues.

Mindfulness is one way of activating the body's natural calming response. This is the "off" switch for the stress reaction cycle, and the "on" switch for all the body's growth and development systems. It can be activated naturally as the body comes back to a place of balance, or we can foster it deliberately. Dr. Herbert Benson, director emeritus of the Benson-Henry Institute for Mind Body Medicine at Massachusetts General Hospital, recommends practicing mindfulness meditation for 20 minutes during the day in order to make it easier to evoke the calming response at night.

## LETTING GO OF THE NARRATIVE

Getting stuck in thinking or rumination is often a factor in preventing sleep. We can't turn off our brain, and it continues to race into the future or gets stuck in the past, going over and over events or experiences. All this can keep us awake. Often the original worry is compounded as we judge or become anxious about it (I shouldn't be so worked up about this/Why can't I stop this?) or about not sleeping (I'm going to be shattered tomorrow if I don't get to sleep soon), and these may be accompanied by uncomfortable physical sensations and tension.

Through regular meditation practice, we begin to see that we are always creating stories about what we are experiencing, and that these stories are influenced by the mood we are in. If we are feeling happy, we will put a positive spin on what is arising, but if we are feeling stressed or down, we are more likely to interpret things negatively; we will even actively look for evidence to corroborate the negative story and discount any evidence to the contrary. Through practicing mindfulness we can learn to see these stories as just that—fairy tales, rather than facts. Once we realize that our thoughts are closely tied to our moods, the power they have over us weakens and we learn to choose where we want to place our attention. This is particularly helpful when we are having trouble sleeping, and we can notice and acknowledge that we are catastrophizing and intentionally bring our attention back to the body, noticing what sensations are arising both internally and externally.

Cultivating attitudes of kindness and non-judging when we meditate encourages us to let go of blaming ourselves and practice self-kindness instead.

## COMING INTO THE BODY

When we practice mindfulness, we are not trying to stop thinking or empty our mind. Instead, we practice diverting our attention from thoughts when we meditate (all thoughts—not just the unhelpful ones), and coming back to a focus such as the breath or the body. Paying attention to changing sensations of the breath or body brings us into the present moment, away from thinking about past or future. We can't be thinking at the same time as being curious about physical sensations. Of course, our attention will be pulled away again, but the encouragement is simply to bring it back to the breath and/or the body. By doing this over and over again we become better able to notice when the mind wanders, and we become more attuned to the body and its sensations.

Over time, many of us become removed from the physical body; perhaps we don't like the way it looks or the way it is aging, or maybe we experience physical pain or discomfort. We end up spending most of our time thinking about our experience, rather than actually experiencing it. Reacquainting ourselves with the body through practicing mindfulness is a way of becoming whole once more: one mind and body. The more familiar we are with the body, the more likely we are to pick up early signs that things aren't quite right.

## BECOMING MORE RESPONSIVE

When we meditate, we quickly become familiar with things not being as we would like them to be. We want to sit still, but suddenly there is an itch on our nose or a fly buzzing about our ear. The automatic reaction is to scratch the itch or swat the fly, but instead we are encouraged to notice the physical sensations and be curious about them, perhaps becoming aware of tension in the body, a stinging sensation, the urge to move ... We notice and name what is arising and how it changes, perhaps getting worse, perhaps fading away. If we do decide to "scratch the itch," we make it a conscious decision and then bring the action of scratching into awareness. Every time we inhibit the automatic unconscious reaction and consciously choose to respond in a different way, we are laying down new patterns of behavior and breaking the chain of reactivity.

## WANTING TO HELP OURSELVES

Practicing mindfulness is a way of learning to take better care of ourselves mentally and physically. As we start paying attention to the way we live our lives, we start noticing the actions and behavior that are helpful and those that are unhelpful. Once we become aware of this, we usually find ourselves intentionally choosing to do more of the helpful and less of the unhelpful. This can be particularly useful when it comes to our own sleep habits. Making some simple changes can create small shifts, each contributing to an overall improvement. However, we are all different, so I would encourage a sense of experimentation and exploration about what you notice about your own habits and behavior, and how they support or affect your sleep quality.

## WAKING UP TO OUR LIVES

The awareness that arises from practicing mindfulness is often described as feeling alert and alive—the opposite of sleepiness. Therefore practicing mindfulness regularly may increase our awareness to a degree that we literally feel more "awake" during the day.

# HELPFUL ATTITUDES

When we practice mindfulness, we consciously cultivate particular attitudes in the way we pay attention to our experience. These attitudes also arise from the meditation practices.

- **Non-striving** We often have a goal in mind—we "should" be able to fall asleep instantly, or we "should" be able to stop worrying or sleep for 8 hours. When we are striving for an outcome, we constantly measure and judge ourselves according to how well or badly we think we are doing. This is unhelpful, and sets us up for disappointment and frustration. It is counterproductive to try to force ourselves to sleep (it will only increase anxiety and tension); instead, we simply focus on our experience in the present moment.

- **Letting go** Being willing to let go of wanting to fix or change our experience (often to make it better) and instead acknowledge how it is (even if we don't like it) is the first step in accepting things as they are. Being willing to let things unfold requires us to let go of wanting to control our experience. Falling asleep requires us to let go of effort and striving.

- **Acceptance** This is an active state of acknowledging how things actually are rather than resisting them or pushing them away (our usual mode). Resisting the way things are takes a lot of energy, and usually involves blaming ourselves, others, or a particular situation. If we can drop the stories we are telling ourselves about "not sleeping" that are fueling our anxiety, we are left with simply being awake. If we are awake, it is better to accept that we are not sleepy, and get up and do something pleasurable or satisfying.

- **Trust** This is tied very closely to non-striving, cultivating a willingness to give it a go as best you can for a reasonable period (several weeks is recommended). Change takes time and doesn't follow a straight trajectory of improvement. Some nights we might sleep worse than others, but that doesn't mean it will last forever. The body is primed to self-regulate, and if we can support those systems with good habits, the body will find its natural rhythm.

- **Patience** We are working with patterns that we have built up over many years, and it takes time to learn to relate to things differently. It's not helpful to expect perfection— we must just do the best we can considering our circumstances. Change often comes about through making small alterations to our lives, each one influencing the next, and even sleeping an extra hour or not creating additional suffering by worrying about being awake can transform how we are feeling.

- **Curiosity** When we are curious, we are interested and we want to find out more; to do that, we must pay attention and move in closer. It seems counterintuitive to move toward something that we don't like or that we see as a threat, but changing the way we perceive our experience is crucial. By consciously moving toward things, we learn to become less reactive and better able to respond to whatever is occurring. By becoming interested in our experience (thoughts, emotions, physical sensations, and behavior), we notice what is present and let go of the need to know why.

- **Beginner's mind** Very often we have a fixed idea about the way something will be, and we see things through our own filters of memory and experience. This saps the vitality from everyday living, since we are not open to seeing what is actually there. If we can bring the fresh eyes of a beginner or child to our experience, we discover all kinds of things. We can apply this to sleep by approaching each night free of the expectations or emotions that are the result of the previous night.

- **Non-judging** When we start noticing our thoughts, we realize that we are judging ourselves, others, and our experience all the time. It is easy to get stuck on thinking that we should be sleeping for a particular number of hours, but it is more helpful simply to acknowledge where we are right now. Being more flexible about how we view sleep will help us to relax, and that creates more conducive conditions for sleep to arise.

- **Kindness** Noticing that internal critical voice and practicing kindness toward ourselves, our experience, and others is fundamental to mindfulness, particularly if we are feeling tired and frustrated from broken nights. Nourish yourself mentally and physically by consciously being kind to yourself.

The practices in Chapter 3 explore ways of cultivating some of these helpful attitudes, which support allowing things to be as they are. As we practice regularly, we gradually find that we become less reactive and better able to respond to whatever is occurring.

We can also consciously apply these attitudes to our sleep routine and the way we approach it (see pages 97–98).

## Changing the brain

Through looking at brain scans of participants before and after an 8-week mindfulness course, neuroscientists discovered an increase in activity in areas of the brain to do with compassion, empathy, and perspective-taking (that is, seeing alternative viewpoints and being less rigid in our thinking), among others. That suggests that these qualities can be improved measurably over a relatively short period of time. We will look at this in more detail on pages 53–55.

# MINDFULNESS: THE RESEARCH

**Interventions based on mindfulness have consistently been shown to reduce perceived stress, rumination or getting stuck in thinking, and physiological symptoms. They have also been shown to improve positive outlook, attention, empathy, self-compassion, and overall quality of life.**

The neuroscience studies mentioned opposite showed changes in the brain that support these self-reported improvements. Increased activity was seen in the areas of the brain to do with focus, attention, perspective-taking, compassion, and empathy, and in the part responsible for more effective regulation of emotions, as well as the pons area of the brainstem, where the REM cycle is regulated and maintained; and there was reduced activity in the amygdala (which activates the stress reaction cycle; see page 46).

## MINDFULNESS AND SLEEP

Research into mindfulness and sleep specifically is still in its infancy, but, since difficulties with sleeping are so often tied to physical and psychological problems, sleep has often been measured as part of studies into mindfulness and conditions such as stress, depression, anxiety, and cancer.

This research suggests that people's subjective sleep quality improves through practicing mindfulness meditation. Subjective sleep quality is acknowledged as an important factor in our perceived quality of life and overall health.

We have already seen that subjective sleep quality is people's perception of how quickly they have fallen asleep, its duration, and how rested they feel on awakening, rather than objective measurements taken in laboratory conditions while the subject cycles through the proper stages of n-REM and REM sleep (see pages 14–17). Two people can have sleep of similar duration with a similar number and length of awakenings, yet rate their sleep quality very differently. This suggests that if we can change the way we relate to our sleep, we can change our perception of it—and that may in turn improve our subjective sleep quality. Mindfulness can help us to do this.

People who experience insomnia often relate to it in a particular way. Understandably, they become absorbed in it as a problem to be fixed, focusing on specific nighttime routines and feeling that they need a specific number of hours' sleep (usually the "official" 8 hours). This lack of flexibility can feed anxiety about sleep. Mindfulness can help us to let go of needing things to be a particular way, and, paradoxically, this willingness to be with things as they are (in this instance awake, or not asleep) creates the right conditions for us to get to where we want to be: a reduction in the anxiety that fuels the wakefulness and that makes us feel miserable and frustrated while we are awake.

Take a moment now to reflect on how you perceive sleep. What routines do you employ to try to ensure you get a good night's sleep? How much sleep do you consider that you need?

How you perceive difficulties with sleeping will determine the severity of your problem. If you see not sleeping as a major problem, you will likely become even more awake and more anxious about sleeping, which will further disrupt your sleep. However, be careful: This is not a reason to blame yourself more. Simply noticing the way we think influences us on many different levels, so congratulate yourself for taking the first steps in learning a different way of relating to sleep.

Often what keeps people awake is thinking—we are unable to switch off—and mindfulness has been shown to be particularly useful in breaking the cycle of rumination and thereby reducing anxiety. We can also help ourselves by taking steps to modify our behavior (see page 36).

While there are recognized limitations in the studies into mindfulness and sleep, and more research is needed, the fact that insomnia, pain, and psychological distress are usually intertwined suggests that an overarching, mindfulness-based approach to sleep problems may help. There is already plenty of accepted evidence for mindfulness-based approaches to chronic pain, anxiety, the prevention of relapse of depression, and other psychological and physical conditions.

# MINDFULNESS-BASED THERAPY FOR INSOMNIA (MBTI)

This relatively new mindfulness-based approach to insomnia has been developed by the psychologist Dr. Jason Ong and his colleagues. Based on Mindfulness-based Stress Reduction (MBSR) and Mindfulness-based Cognitive Therapy (MBCT), it includes regular meditation practice as well as specific behavioral components including stimulus control (only going to bed when you feel sleepy), sleep restriction (following a schedule of going to bed and rising that is less than usual, thereby increasing the appetite for sleep), and good sleep hygiene (see page 36). The emphasis is on changing your relationship to sleep, rather than focusing on the amount of sleep you achieve each night. Dr. Ong stresses that it takes time, discipline, and consistency to follow this approach.

## Mindfulness and sleep studies

One study (Hubbling et al., 2014), which looked specifically at whether a mindfulness course could help with chronic insomnia, found that although participants didn't sleep more than before, they reported sleeping better and waking more refreshed. Overall they felt less distressed about their insomnia and better able to cope when it arose. As well as meditating regularly, the group practiced yoga, which helped them to feel more flexible and reduced aches and pains. Overall they felt calmer and less stressed during the day (and they noted the reverse when they didn't practice mindfulness meditation). The increased awareness they gained through practice, as well as greater curiosity and openness, led them to make conscious decisions about their sleep routines, making good sleep hygiene a priority. Letting go of striving for a particular outcome (sleep), and cultivating a willingness to accept the present moment as it is, gave participants the confidence to cope with whatever arose, even occasional recurrences of insomnia.

Another study (Carlson and Garland, 2005) on the benefits of MBSR on sleep, mood, stress, and fatigue in cancer patients found that reported sleep quality improved and stress, mood disturbance, and fatigue decreased.

In both these studies, the support of others in the research group contributed to the positive results for participants.

# CHAPTER 3
# THE PRACTICES

This chapter suggests a range of meditation practices and activities to cultivate helpful skills and help to establish a regular mindfulness practice, with a mixture of formal and informal practices. See pages 41–44 to learn about the difference, as well as for some tips on how to make the most of your practice.

By practicing regularly during the day, we reduce our overall stress as well as introducing other benefits (see page 53) that usually help to improve the quality of our sleep. Some practices are designed to cultivate particular qualities and attitudes that are helpful overall when you are faced with things not being as you would like. There are also some practices that can be done if you are awake in the night or having trouble falling asleep. Just remember that it is important not to do them with the expectation that they will send you to sleep.

Remember to take care of yourself at all times, and stop if any practice feels uncomfortable or causes pain. We are not trying to cultivate any particular experience when we meditate, so there is no expectation that it should be a particularly enjoyable experience—the important thing is to show up to yourself and do it regardless!

It is your choice which practices to do when, but if you are new to meditation I would encourage you to start with Paying Attention to the Breath on page 61 or Paying Attention to the Body on page 71. These build helpful foundational skills.

# CHECKING YOUR POSTURE

When we are doing a more formal sitting practice, it is helpful to take a moment to pay attention to how we are sitting, since our posture can support or undermine our frame of mind. For example, if we are slouched and hunched, with our head falling forward, our mind is more likely to be sleepy and contracted. Sitting up straight in a way that is alert, open, and relaxed will encourage our attention in the same way.

Sitting is only one option, however, and many of the practices in this book can be done lying down. Just be aware that lying down might encourage you to fall asleep (which, of course, may be just what you want—but remember that we are not meditating in order to fall asleep). Also included here is guidance for checking your posture when standing (for example, if you are doing a walking meditation).

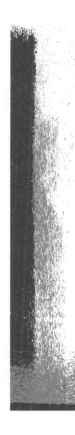

## SITTING PRACTICE

Follow these steps whenever the instructions are "check your posture" for a seated practice.

- Use a kitchen or dining chair rather than a soft easy chair.

- Experiment with keeping your eyes open or closed. If you have them open, drop your gaze to the floor a little in front of you and keep your gaze soft and unfocused.

- Place both feet flat on the floor to encourage a sense of being grounded. Support them with a pillow if necessary.

- Have your hands in a supported position: Cupped in your lap or palms of the hands resting on your thighs.

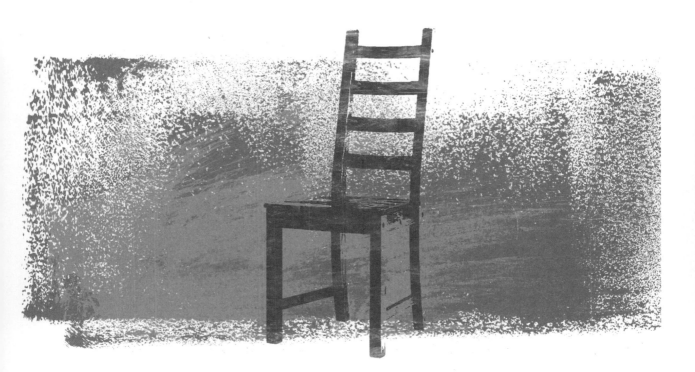

1. Run your attention up from the soles of the feet, through the ankles, lower legs, knees, and thighs. When you reach the pelvis, experiment with rocking it slightly forward or letting it roll backward. **What do you notice?** When the pelvis is tilted forward, it encourages the torso to lift out of the pelvis. When it rolls backward, the spine collapses and so does our pose.

2. Take your attention into the base of the spine, and in your mind's eye slowly run it up the spine, vertebra by vertebra, through the lower back, middle back, upper back, and shoulders, into the neck and skull, and out through the top of the head. Imagine the top of the head lifting very slightly so the chin tucks in.

3. From time to time during any practice, **check in and adjust your posture as necessary**—particularly if you are feeling sleepy.

## LYING-DOWN PRACTICE

1   If you are lying down to meditate, lie flat on your back with your legs outstretched and your arms by your side (or place your hands palms down on your belly). You can place a pillow or bolster under your knees or lower back for additional support, if you like.

2   Take a moment to **tune into any parts of the body that are in contact with the surface on which you are lying.** Perhaps take a deep breath and then let it go, letting the body relax into the supporting surface.

## STANDING IN MOUNTAIN PRACTICE

1   Bring yourself to an upright, balanced position with both feet flat on the floor.

2   In your mind's eye, drop your attention to the soles of the feet and then slowly move the awareness up through the feet, ankles, lower legs, knees, thighs, hips, and into the buttocks and torso.

3   Tiptoe your attention up from the base of the spine, through the lower back, middle back, upper back, and shoulders, and through the neck and crown of the head. Standing tall, standing firm—**standing like a mountain.**

### OTHER OPTIONS

If you want to sit cross-legged on the floor, make sure your hips are positioned higher than your knees. You can sit on a yoga block, pillow, or small stack of books to achieve this. Your knees should be supported, so if they are shooting up to the ceiling place pillows underneath.

# PAYING ATTENTION TO THE BREATH

The breath is a great object to focus our attention on: It is accessible and, because it is a moving target, we must exert some effort to keep paying attention to it. The breath also changes according to our frame of mind. If we are anxious or scared, we may find ourselves breathing faster and shallower or perhaps even holding the breath, whereas when we are relaxed we usually breathe more slowly and deeply.

How is your breath right now? Simply drop your attention into the chest or belly and begin to notice it, becoming aware of its characteristics. There is no need to change it or breathe in a particular way (such as inhaling and exhaling through the nose instead of the mouth, or vice versa). By tuning into the breath regularly, we can become familiar with our "normal" state and any patterns that may arise according to how we are feeling.

We can also do this as a more formal meditation practice by following the steps described on the following pages.

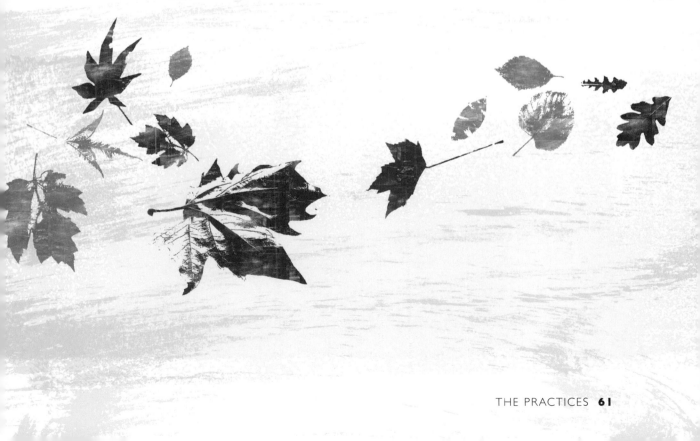

## THE PRACTICE

1   Find a place where you won't be disturbed and check your posture (see page 58). Begin by **becoming aware of the breath**. Where are you feeling it most strongly? This may be in the belly, in the chest, or around the nostrils or upper lip. It doesn't matter where it is, but make a clear intention to place your attention there. You may want to place a hand on the belly to help connect with the felt sense of breathing.

2   Continue following the breath. Be curious about it. **What does it feel like physically in the body?** Notice the in-breath, stay with it, and then notice the transition to an out-breath, and then back to an in-breath.

3   Sooner rather than later you will find that your attention is somewhere else—maybe thinking about what you have to do, about a vacation, or about another person. It is the nature of the mind to wander, and all you have to do is **acknowledge it and redirect your attention** back to the breath. You will find yourself doing this over and over again, and that's okay.

4   Every time you realize your attention has wandered, you are experiencing a moment of **awareness**. Every time you bring your attention back with an attitude of **kindness** and **gentleness**, you are cultivating those qualities toward yourself. It is also helpful to notice what is on your mind, simply as feedback. What is grabbing your attention?

5   Begin by doing this for 5 minutes or so, then gradually extend the time if you can.

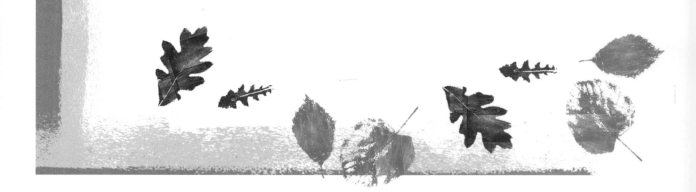

## SOME THINGS TO BE AWARE OF DURING MEDITATION

- We are not trying to empty our mind or stop thinking. Instead, we are learning to let go of thinking and choose where we want to place our attention. We are also learning more about our mind and where it goes

- A busy mind is an opportunity to lay down and reinforce new neural pathways in the brain. You must bring your attention back repeatedly for change to happen.

- Notice if you have a tendency to give yourself a hard time about having a busy mind or even about particular thoughts that arise. Remember that we are practicing paying attention with kindness and open-heartedness, and without judging. There's no need to judge yourself for judging, either! Simply notice: Ah, there I go again.

- We are not trying to achieve a particular state of mind. Your mind may settle or you may simply notice how strong the urge to get on with "doing" is. Whatever arises is simply your experience. We are not striving for any particular experience.

### OTHER OPTIONS

Sometimes people find paying attention to the breath a bit tricky, and it can make you feel a little panicky. If that happens, experiment with Paying Attention to the Body (see page 71) or Breathing Through Soles of the Feet (see page 67) instead. From time to time, experiment with tuning into the breath toward the end of one of these practices, and notice how that feels. If it feels okay, continue; if not, it's fine to simply stay with the body.

## PRACTICING WHEN YOU ARE OUT AND ABOUT

You can also do this practice more informally, perhaps while sitting on a bus or train, or at your desk. You can do it standing up or lying down. Practice doing it as often as you can in a variety of situations and locations, including at night.

# COUNTING BREATHS

The traditional suggestion for getting to sleep was to try counting sheep. This practice works in a similar way—if the mind is particularly busy, we can count our breaths as a way of steadying our attention and moving our attention out of the head (thinking) and into the body.

In this practice, we count up to ten and then start again. When you find yourself going beyond 10, simply start again at 1. You can do this practice lying in bed or sitting in the same way as Paying Attention to the Breath on pages 61–62.

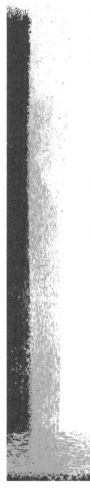

## THE PRACTICE

1 Whether sitting or lying down, check your posture (see page 58). **Begin to tune into your breathing.** Notice how the breath is made up of an in-breath and an out-breath. For counting purposes, both of these make up one whole breath.

2 Every time you breathe in and out, count 1. Continue up to 10 and then start again.

3 **Don't worry if you lose count or go beyond 10.** As soon as you realize, simply return to 1. Continue for as long or short a time as you like.

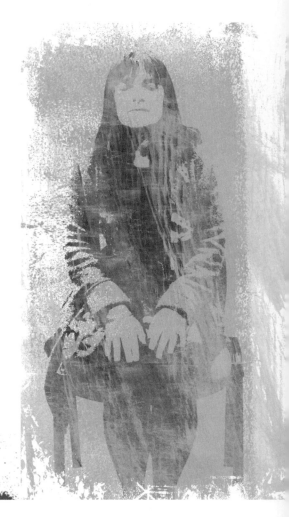

# LETTING GO INTO THE OUT-BREATH

**This is a good practice to do lying down, perhaps before you fall asleep or if you wake in the night.**

Remember that whenever we do these practices, we are not doing them with a particular outcome in mind—you may fall asleep, but also you may not, and that's okay. If you expect to fall asleep and then don't, you will most likely feel frustrated, disappointed, and more, and that is counterproductive. It will only fuel anxiety, which will feed the wakefulness.

## THE PRACTICE

1   If you are doing this lying down, **begin by becoming aware of the whole body**. Notice where it is in contact with the bed or mat and how that feels—soft? Hard? (You can do the practice sitting if you prefer.)

2   Take a deep breath in and let it out suddenly (if you make a noise as you exhale, that's okay). Do this two or three times, noticing as you do so **how the body softens and lets go** as you breathe out.

3   Then begin tuning into the out-breath. Notice how the body relaxes and softens—perhaps **be curious** about which parts of the body feel loose. Just let go.

4   You may notice a feeling of "holding on" or tension in a particular part of the body, perhaps in the face or the torso. Simply **acknowledge that tension is here.** You may experience a letting go, but there is no need to force anything.

5   Every time the mind wanders, bring it back (see Paying Attention to the Breath, page 61).

# BREATH AND MOVEMENT

We can tune into the breath and body simultaneously by connecting the two—moving in time with our breathing. This practice employs small movements of the hands.

This practice can be done sitting or lying down, and the type of movement is less important than synchronizing it as best you can with the in- and out-breath.

## THE PRACTICE

1  Whether sitting or lying down, **check your posture** (see page 58). Your eyes can be open or closed.

2  Take a moment to connect with any areas of the body that are in contact with the surface that is supporting you. This may be the bed, chair, or floor. **Notice and be curious about how that contact feels**—its texture (rough, smooth, hard, soft …) and maybe its temperature.

3  Place your hands on the belly and **become aware of any physical sensations**. Notice how the hands move in response to the rise and fall of the belly as the breath enters and leaves the body.

4  **Expand your attention** to include the sensations of breathing. Then expand further to become aware of the hands.

5  When you feel ready, **begin moving the hands in response to the breath.** You might open out the hands as you breathe in, then, as the in-breath turns into an out-breath, let the palms float toward the belly. Repeat as you breathe out once more, and continue in this way for as long as you wish.

6  Remember that it is normal for your attention to be pulled away. All you need to do is acknowledge that "thinking" and **bring the attention back to the hands**, moving in time to your breath.

# BREATHING THROUGH THE SOLES OF THE FEET

We can use the breath as a vehicle for our attention—directing it into and out of different parts of the body (the Body Scan on page 68 is a great way to practice this). In this practice, we drop our attention to the soles of the feet and imagine that we are breathing in and out from there.

When you are sitting or standing and the soles of the feet are in contact with the floor, this practice can feel very grounding. This can be helpful if you are feeling anxious or panicky. Breathing through the Soles of the Feet is a good alternative to Paying Attention to the Breath (see page 61), if focusing on your breathing feels a bit tricky or uncomfortable.

## THE PRACTICE

1   Check your posture (see page 58). Then, narrowing your focus to the breath, tune into the in- and out-breath.

2   Direct your attention to the soles of the feet and become aware of their contact with the ground. Then, as you breathe in, **imagine that the breath is entering the body through the feet**, sweeping up through the body, filling it with oxygen and life. As you breathe out, the breath is leaving the body through the soles of the feet, cleansing the body.

3   Continue in this way, breathing in and out and imagining the breath sweeping in and out through the soles of the feet, for as long as you like.

4   You might find that you get stuck on wondering "Am I doing this right?" There is no right or wrong—it's simply about **having a sense of the whole body breathing** at the same time as connecting to the earth beneath you.

# BODY SCAN

**The Body Scan is a lying-down practice, and although the intention is "to fall awake," people often find themselves falling asleep while doing it—which can be helpful if you are having trouble sleeping.**

If you tend to fall asleep while doing it and want to encourage that, Jon Kabat-Zinn (author of *Full Catastrophe Living*, 1990) recommends doing this practice at bedtime or during the night, but also at another time during the day and at that time making a clear intention to stay awake. However, if you are doing it in bed, it is always best to let go of any expectations of a particular outcome. Even if the practice helps you to fall asleep one night, it may have a very different effect the next, and that is normal.

## THINGS TO REMEMBER

While doing the Body Scan, keep the following points in mind:

- As soon as you realize that your attention has wandered (and it will), simply bring it back to the body without any judgment.
- We are not expecting any particular outcome, such as to feel relaxed or to fall asleep. Sometimes that will happen, but other times it will not.
- Each time you do this, practice beginner's mind (see page 51) and the curiosity that comes with it. Imagine you know nothing about this body or how it feels. What do you discover? You may notice sensations in some parts of the body but not in others, or perhaps no sensations at all. We are not interested in analyzing why this is, but simply in bringing awareness to it.
- We can store emotions and trauma in the body, and sometimes these may be released through tears or sadness. However, if the practice feels uncomfortable for you at any time, please stop immediately.
- Don't worry about the order in which you do the different parts of the body. The important thing is simply to tune into it.
- If you do fall asleep every time you do this, you may just be chronically tired. Experiment with doing it seated and with your eyes open.

# THE PRACTICE

1   Lie on your back with your legs outstretched and arms by your side. Your eyes can be open or closed. Take a moment to **notice the different parts of the body in contact with the bed or floor.** Perhaps take a deep breath and then exhale loudly, letting the body soften into the surface.

2   Take your attention to the breath in the belly. You can place one hand on the belly to help **connect with the sensations of breathing:** The rise and fall of the belly. This is your home base. At any point in the practice, if you lose your place or things feel a bit tricky, just bring your attention back to the breath in the belly and stay there for as long as you wish.

3   Place your hand back at your side and move your attention from the torso down through the left leg into the left foot. Pay attention to the toes on your left foot. Is there anything to notice? Any numbness, tingling, itchiness, textile touching skin, warmth or coolness …? We are not looking for anything in particular, but rather **noticing what is present (or absent).** If you don't feel anything at all, that's okay.

4   Move your attention from the toes to the sole of the left foot, the heel, the top of the foot, and then the foot as a whole, all the time noticing whatever is arising or present. **Be curious about what your experience is right now.**

5   Take your attention to your breath, and in your mind's eye imagine that you are directing the breath into and out of the left foot, as if the left foot were breathing. Continue for a few moments.

6   Let go of the left foot, move your attention to the lower left leg, and explore this in the same way.

7   Move up through the left leg and then, taking your attention to the breath, imagine that you are breathing in and out, up and down the length of the left leg.

8 Continue in this way round the whole body. You can do individual elements such as fingers, or divide the body into sections. Explore the back of the torso and the front, as well as the neck (and internal throat) and the head, including the skull, individual features, and the face as a whole.

9 When you have finished scanning the whole body, **take your attention to the breath once more** and imagine that you are breathing in through the soles of the feet and out through the top of the head. Let the breath sweep from one end of the body to the other for a couple of minutes.

10 End by **becoming aware of the body as a whole** in contact with the surface.

## OTHER OPTIONS

If you have limited time and it feels too much to do the entire body, why not simply focus on a small area, such as the hand? Explore individual fingers, the spaces between them, the thumb, the palm, the back of the hand. You can do just one hand, or try doing both and noticing the differences and similarities between them.

# PAYING ATTENTION TO THE BODY

**Most of us spend much of our lives in our heads. We are disconnected from the body and sometimes have an uneasy relationship with it. Perhaps it is aging and letting us down physically, or it doesn't look the way we think it should; maybe it gives us pain or limits what we can do. Practices such as this one give us an opportunity to become reacquainted with the body.**

It is interesting to notice what happens when you turn your attention to the body. What do you discover? We notice physical sensations, and—importantly—how we relate to them. We usually soften around those we like and tense up around those we don't. This tension can create secondary discomfort as well as physiological problems in the longer term.

In this practice, we begin to learn different ways to respond to physical sensations. We practice with the irritating itch or pins and needles to learn how to be with more serious discomfort if that arises. Practicing being with discomfort is an important first step in learning to allow and accept our experience, rather than trying to get rid of it. There are always going to be experiences in life that we don't like, but we can learn to live with them.

There are certain familiar themes that are key to this practice. Try to keep them in mind before you begin:

KINDNESS It is important that there is a strong element of kindness and gentleness in this practice. There is no point in gritting our teeth and determinedly staying with discomfort. That is the opposite of mindfulness. Instead, we are more interested in moving a little closer to areas of discomfort and hovering around them as we explore them, but pulling back to the anchor of the breath as often as we need to.

THE WANDERING MIND You will find that your attention is always being pulled away from the body into thinking, whether it is about the sensations or about other things or other people, in the past or the future. Whenever you become aware of this, simply acknowledge it and bring your attention gently back to the body. We do this over and over again.

THE JUDGING MIND We may notice that we start giving ourselves a hard time: "I should be doing this better." "Come on, it's not rocket science—keep focusing!" That is normal. We acknowledge it—judging is here—and then bring our attention back with a huge dollop of kindness.

Meditating in this way, whether our focus is the breath, the body, sounds, or something else, shines a light on what goes on in the mind. We notice habitual patterns of thinking and attitudes to ourselves and others. This is all useful feedback. We can start doing something different only once we have become aware of what we might want to change.

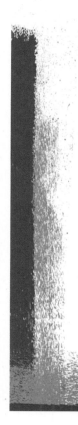

## THE PRACTICE

1  This is traditionally a sitting practice, but you could do it lying down. Either way, begin by checking your posture (see page 58). Bring your attention to the breath. **Where do you notice it most strongly?** It may be in the belly or the chest, or around the nostrils and upper lip. It doesn't matter where, but just choose and **make that the focus of your attention**. Stay with the breath for a few minutes, bringing the attention back when it wanders. (For more detailed instructions on how to pay attention to the breath, see page 61.)

2  Expand the attention to include the whole body. Perhaps notice first of all any areas that are in contact with another surface—this may be a chair, bed, textile, skin … Explore how that feels in terms of **texture, temperature, and sensation**, noticing differences and similarities. Become aware of how

you relate to whatever is arising—is it pleasurable or unpleasant? Perhaps it is neutral. Simply notice how that manifests in the body.

3   Notice if there are any parts of the body that begin calling for attention. Be curious about any sensation that is present, and try to discover a bit more about it. Where exactly is it? Is it solid or insubstantial? Is it moving or fixed? What kind of shape does the sensation have? How would you describe it: tingling, stabbing, throbbing, needling …? As long as it feels okay, move your attention in a little closer. We often use the analogy of getting to know someone new, and we want to have a similar attitude of **curiosity and interest** here, rather than one of analyzing why we might be feeling a particular way.

4   We can also direct the breath, targeting the sensation itself and imagining that we are breathing into and out of that particular area. We are not trying to get rid of the sensation, but practicing a different way of being with it— **allowing it to be present**.

5   If a sensation is particularly strong, it can be helpful to turn the attention to the breath (where you started) and hang out there, occasionally tuning into the physical sensation for a moment or two but returning to the anchor of the breath if necessary. However, **taking care of yourself is always the priority**, so stop at any time if necessary.

6   We can also move, adjusting our position or "scratching the itch." Ideally, **we make a conscious choice to do this** and then move with awareness, knowing what we are doing as we are doing it. This is the opposite of the usual automatic scratching or fidgeting that we do unconsciously to get rid of an uncomfortable sensation.

7   Continue for as long as you wish, then narrow your attention to the breath for a moment or two before finishing.

# OUTLINING THE BODY

When we are lying awake, it is very easy to become caught up in a thought spiral about not sleeping: Why we can't sleep, how it's affecting us, and all the associated emotions these thoughts create. It is helpful if we can shift from a sense of needing to do something about not being able to sleep, to practicing simply being as we are—which, in this moment, is awake. We can do this by making the body our focus. This might be a part of the body, such as the breath (see page 61), or the body as a whole (see page 71), or, as here, an exploration of the outline of the body in two and three dimensions.

Although this is a lying-down practice, remember to let go of any expectation that you will fall asleep.

# THE PRACTICE

1    In your mind's eye, **begin outlining the body**, as if you were drawing around it. Then begin moving your attention across the contours of the body three-dimensionally, for example around and across the top of the feet, the belly, the chest, and the head. Always maintain an awareness of any points of contact with the bed, and mentally draw around them.

2    Notice any physical sensations, such as touch and temperature, or internal sensations, such as tingling or numbness. We are not expecting to feel anything in particular, or to have a specific experience. We are simply **connecting with this body lying here in this moment**.

3    Every time you become aware of the mind wandering, acknowledge it as "thinking" and **gently bring your attention back** to outlining the body. We do this over and over again. It is the nature of the mind to wander, and we are training ourselves to notice it wandering and bring it back to a focus, in this case the body. It is important that you don't give yourself a hard time when your mind wanders. We can't stop thinking, but we can learn to choose where we want to place our attention, whether on our thoughts or on the body. In this practice, we are choosing always to bring our attention back to the body.

4    Continue in this way as long as you wish. You may fall asleep, or you may "fall awake." **There is no goal**, and if you strive for a particular outcome you are setting yourself up for failure.

# JUST THREE THINGS

When we begin practicing mindfulness, we soon learn how helpful it is to turn our attention to the body. By cultivating an attitude of curiosity about what is arising physically in the body, we are able to shift our attention from our head, which is often busy overthinking the latest drama in our lives. There are many body-focused practices to explore; this one is particularly simple and therefore ideal if you are lying awake in bed. Just accept whatever happens. You may fall asleep, and you may not. The intention is simply to be present to whatever arises moment by moment.

In this practice we focus our attention on just three things, one after the other: Temperature, touch, and breath.

## THE PRACTICE

1 Lie flat on your back with your legs outstretched, your feet falling away, and your arms at your side a little away from the body. Turn your hands palm up.

2 **TEMPERATURE:** Notice any part of the body that feels warm, whether externally or internally, and **explore what the felt sensation of warmth is like.** Can you notice different degrees of warmth? Is there a point at which warm becomes hot? Notice how you are responding to what you find—does it feel positive, negative, or neutral (we are not looking for a specific response, simply noticing the fact that we always judge our experience to some degree).

3 Let go of warmth, and now notice any part of the body that feels cool or cold. Explore internally and externally in the same way as for warmth and heat, again **noticing how you respond.**

4   **TOUCH:** Letting go of temperature, turn your attention to touch. Notice any points of contact with the mattress (the heels, the backs of the calves, the thighs, the buttocks ...). **Notice how the contact actually feels** (hard, soft, welcoming, resisting ...). What else is touching: Fabric in contact with skin, skin on skin ... how many different types of contact can you identify? Explore touch.

5   **BREATH:** Letting go of touch, narrow your attention to focus solely on your breathing. Notice where you feel it most strongly. Perhaps notice if it is slow and deep, or short and shallow, or if it varies. There is no need to change your breathing or try to breathe in a particular way; **simply allow the breath to breathe itself.** Become aware of your breathing. You might begin by focusing on the part of the body where you feel the breath most strongly (the chest or belly), but as your attention becomes focused, notice where else in the body you are experiencing breathing. Become aware of movement, rhythm, rising, falling, expanding, contracting ...

6   When you are ready, **expand your attention to include the whole body,** noticing the temperature, any sensations of touch, and the breath entering and leaving this body.

## TRY THIS

If you are struggling to understand the difference between thinking about the breath and becoming aware of the breath, try this exercise by mindfulness teacher Michael Chaskalson. First, turn your attention to your hand and begin thinking about it. Perhaps notice what it looks like, what it is capable of. This is thinking. Then clap both hands together vigorously for a moment or so. Become aware of any physical sensations arising: How they feel, where they are, how they change ... You are simply aware of physical sensations. Can you see the difference between the two?

# A MORNING WALK AS PRACTICE

The dark of night and light of day are determined by the Earth's rotation around the sun, and our sleep cycle, regulated by the circadian rhythm (see page 18), is closely linked to these natural cycles. Our sleep cycle can easily be disrupted by irregular hours, shift work, and jet lag, as well as physical and psychological conditions. We can help to strengthen or reset a disrupted circadian rhythm by exposing ourselves to light (indoors or out), which will signal to the brain that it is day and time to wake up. A morning walk will energize us and help to reset a disrupted circadian rhythm, and it can also be an opportunity for some mindfulness practice. Do remember the importance of practicing without any particular expectations (see page 50).

Take a walk first thing—it could be on the way to work or simply a stroll through a local park or around the block. To make the walk a practice, walk and know that you are walking. You don't need to walk more slowly than usual, but do pay attention to what is arising. Avoid the temptation to put on your headphones or check your cellphone or email as you are walking.

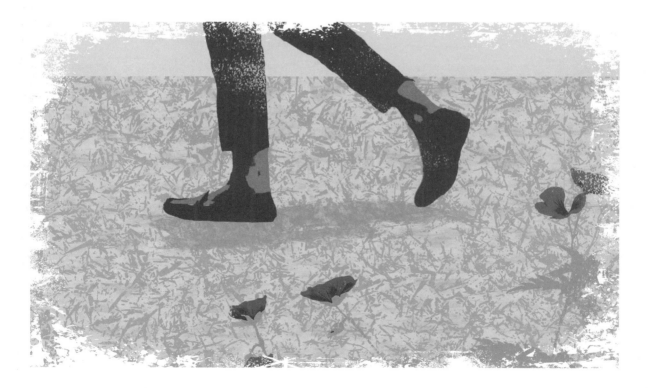

# THE PRACTICE

1   Begin by **dropping your attention to the soles of your feet.** Notice that sense of contact and how the sensations shift as the pressure varies from toe to heel and from one foot to the other.

2   You may choose to **tune into your breathing** as you walk, noticing the in-breath and the out-breath while maintaining awareness of your feet on the ground.

3   After a while, you may want to **expand your attention** to become aware of the rest of the body: The legs, torso, arms, and head. Continue to expand the attention to **become aware of the environment**—the sights, sounds, and smells around you.

4   If you have time and feel comfortable doing so, you may choose **to stop and stand still** (you could do this as you wait to cross a street, for example). Soak up the morning light, perhaps experience a sense of warmth on the body, or of cold air touching the skin. Open up to the sounds of nature—the birdsong or the breeze in the trees—or perhaps the buzz of traffic and people around you.

5   When you are ready, continue walking. This practice can be as long or as short as you wish. **Give yourself the gift of this time for yourself** before you enter the busy-ness of the day ahead.

## OTHER OPTIONS

If you can't go outside, try this practice indoors by walking across a room. Open the drapes, and stand (or sit if that is better for you) and look out the window from time to time, drinking in the early-morning light.

# PRACTICING LETTING GO

When things don't go the way we would like them to, it is easy to become
trapped in a cycle of negative thinking. This avoidance state of mind is when
we don't like the way things are, and we want them to be different. If we don't
think we have slept well, we may catastrophize about the consequences,
perhaps blaming ourselves or others or the environment and wishing it were
different. This activates the body's internal stress reaction (see page 46).
Repeated activation doesn't allow time for the stress hormones, such as
cortisol, to disperse. Cortisol inhibits new neural branching in the brain and
keeps us stuck in negative thinking, and so it goes on.

Even healthy sleepers wake periodically through the night, and that need not affect your
sleep quality. What does affect it is the way you relate to it. Our perception of our
experience can be positive or negative, and that is something we can influence. Even if we
did have a broken night, we are perpetuating and exacerbating the consequences if we
continue to perceive it negatively. We can feed negativity by the words we use to describe
something, or by paying it too much attention.

We all fall into unhelpful patterns of thinking from time to time, particularly if we are
exhausted. However, the more we practice mindful awareness, the more often we will
notice these thoughts as they arise, and it will become possible to see them simply as a
transitory mental event rather than a concrete fact: "Ah, there I go again!"

Letting go of something that we perceive as making us unhappy isn't easy, but it is
possible—this is the part of suffering that is optional in the sense that we are feeding it
through our thoughts and actions, keeping it "live." Breaking this cycle is one way in which
mindfulness has been shown to be particularly helpful.

# THE PRACTICE

1   Begin by paying attention to the way you describe your night's sleep (either to others or simply in your thoughts). Do you catastrophize or over-generalize ("Yet another bad night as usual!"), or something else?

2   Once you have noticed the negative thoughts and acknowledged the pattern (without judging it), turn your attention to the body and **notice how the thoughts and emotions are manifesting physically.** Are you aware of any sensations (perhaps tension or tightening)? Even if you don't notice anything, it is still important to **tune in to the body** with a sense of friendly interest. Name any emotions that you become aware of: You might notice a sense of frustration or irritation with yourself or somebody else.

3   If the emotions and/or sensations are particularly strong, you can direct the breath into and out of the area where they are strongest, or simply settle your attention on the breath in the chest or breathe through the feet on the floor (see page 67).

4   You may notice from time to time through the day that your thoughts return to the previous night and then jump forward to the forthcoming night in nervous anticipation that it will be a repeat. This is normal, and the instruction remains the same: **Notice, acknowledge, and bring your attention to the body and the breath.** Repeat over and over!

5   Remind yourself that each night is a new opportunity for things to be different. We can't change the past and we can't predict the future, but we can **influence the way we respond to what is arising in the present.** We can **choose to be with it,** even if it feels uncomfortable (you might want to read Exploring Resistance; see page 103). We can choose not to stoke our anxiety by turning our attention to something more helpful: The breath and/or the body.

# BEING WITH SOUNDS

Noise can be a big factor in preventing sleep. Whether it's in the early hours or if you are a shift worker trying to sleep during the day, neighbors playing music, roadwork, sirens, or even a ticking clock can feel intrusive when you are trying to fall asleep. Regularly practicing being with sound is a way of building up skills such as exploring your experience with curiosity rather than resistance, and letting go of the narrative we often create around noises and the way they affect us, as well as using the breath and body as an anchor. All these are skills that you can draw on when you are lying in bed awake.

Before doing this for the first time, I recommend practicing Paying Attention to the Breath (see page 61) and Paying Attention to the Body (see page 71) a few times.

When doing the practice, notice:
- Sound as a collection of notes at a particular pitch and timbre.
- How the body responds to a sound. Where do you feel it? How would you describe it?
- How you relate to the sound. Does it appeal to you and draw you in, or do you react against it and try to get rid of it or push it away? Whatever you notice, explore how this actually feels in the body.
- Any emotions that may arise: Frustration, irritation, happiness … Be curious about how an emotion manifests physically in the body.
- When you begin to create a story around a particular sound, such as focusing on how noisy the neighbors are, perhaps imagining that they are deliberately keeping you awake or that you will never get to sleep now and will be exhausted tomorrow … When you realize, simply let it go and return to exploring the physical sense of the sound. You may find it helpful to return to the breath for a time if a story is particularly strong.

Continue in this way for a short time and then bring your attention back to your breath for a few moments before finishing the practice.

Remember that we are not trying to make ourselves like a sound or noise. We are simply exploring how we experience it and noticing how we relate to it, how that feels in the head, heart, and body, and what may arise in terms of action and behavior.

## THE PRACTICE

1  Check your posture (see page 58). Begin by locating the place where you feel the breath most strongly—in the belly or chest, or around the nostrils or upper lip—and making that the focus of your attention. **Keep your attention on the breath as you breathe,** feeling the sensations of the in-breath, the pause as the in-breath becomes an out-breath, and so on. Whenever your mind wanders, bring the attention back to the breath, without judging yourself. Stay with the breath for a few minutes.

2  Then **expand your attention to include the whole body,** noticing anywhere it is in contact with the floor or seat, and becoming aware of any physical sensations. Notice if there is a sense of liking or not liking any of these sensations, and what that feels like. What accompanying sensations do you notice? What thought story is created around such sensations and your reaction to them? Simply notice and acknowledge.

3  When you feel ready, turn your attention to receiving sound. It is as if **your body is a radar,** picking up any sounds that come into your awareness—near or far. Remember the helpful attitudes (see page 50), in particular curiosity, and bring them to bear on your experience.

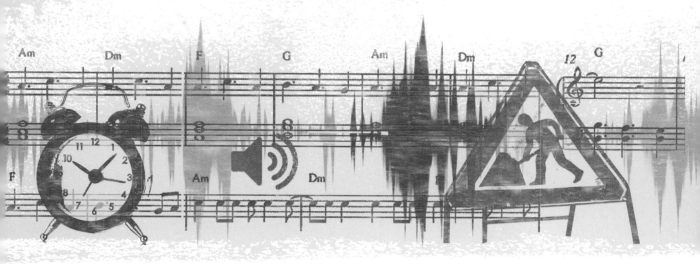

# MINDFUL EATING

How often do you eat while talking to someone, watching television, or checking your cellphone? How does it affect your meal? Do you notice what you are eating—the flavor, texture, smell, and taste? If your attention is distracted, you most likely don't! However, it is very simple to practice something different, and eating mindfully is possible for all of us. It is a straightforward way to move out of the busy-ness of "doing" into "being" present in the moment.

The more familiar the "being" mode becomes, the easier we will find it to consciously switch between the two modes. Incorporating practices such as this one into your everyday life will make it easier for you to switch consciously at night when you can't sleep, for example.

Many people find that this practice makes their food taste more satisfying and also that they eat less, because they recognize the signs of feeling full sooner than they usually do. However, bear in mind that sometimes what we are eating isn't tasty, and bringing that into awareness won't necessarily be pleasant—and that's okay too!

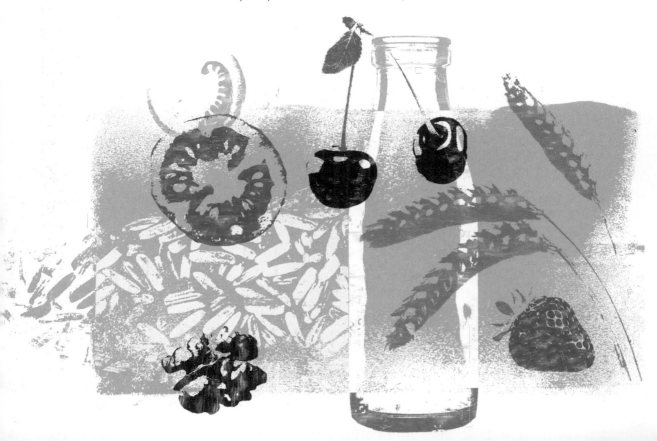

## THE PRACTICE

1   If you are doing this practice for the first time, you may want to try it when you are on your own. You can do it with a single bite, a snack or meal, or a drink (herbal tea is a particularly good option, because of its strong aroma). You may want to **focus simply on the first bite, spoonful, or sip.**

2   There is no particular order or steps to follow. We simply pay attention to what we are eating or drinking, engaging the senses—**sight, smell, taste, touch, and sound**—as we chew, crunch, and swallow. Mindful eating is about **savoring your food and drink.**

3   There is no need to eat or drink more slowly, but doing so can help to remind us that we are **exploring food and drink in a different way from usual.** You may notice that a particular smell or flavor brings a memory into sharp focus, which may have positive associations—or not. Simply notice.

# WALKING WITH NOWHERE TO GO

Rather than lying awake becoming agitated that you are not sleeping, it is a good idea to get up and do something. Walking is an easy movement practice that you can do to shift the attention out of the head and into the body.

You don't need any equipment or to listen to guidance—simply walk and know that you are walking. You don't need a large space, either—perhaps 6 feet (about 2 m), but it can be less. You can walk up and down a corridor or room, or round in a circle. Your arms can be by your sides, or clasped behind or in front of you. It's great to do this barefoot to increase the sensory experience of your feet in contact with the floor, but you can wear shoes if you prefer.

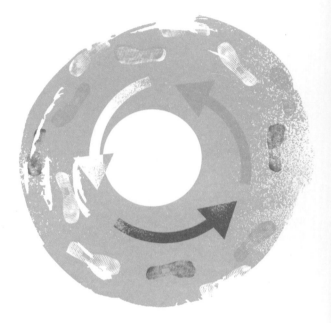

## OTHER OPTIONS

You can of course do this practice during the day. If you struggle to fit in formal practice, use any occasion when you are walking as an opportunity for informal practice. Try it and see.

# THE PRACTICE

1  Begin by standing in mountain (see page 60), running your attention right up through your whole body.

2  Return your attention to the soles of the feet and **notice how the weight is distributed**—is it evenly balanced? Shift your weight over to one side and begin to peel the heel of the opposite foot off the floor (starting with whichever foot feels most natural to you). Notice how **the sensations change as the feeling of pressure eases**, and the foot moves through space before making contact with the floor. Which part comes in contact first?

3  Then notice how the other foot begins to peel off the floor, and so on. Explore **the sense of walking step by step**, keeping the attention on the feet to begin with.

4  If you are walking in a straight line, pause whenever you come to the end. Stand still, then **consciously make the decision to turn**, and do so with awareness. Notice how the distribution of weight may feel unsteady and awkward in that transitional moment, and then how it feels to have a different viewpoint. Continue walking.

5  After a while, expand your attention from the soles of the feet and **become aware of the whole body moving through space**. Perhaps include the environment—its sounds and smells—as well. Then narrow the attention once more to the soles of the feet. Switch back and forth in this way as often as you wish.

6  When you come to an end, take a moment to stand in mountain, as at the start.

# ALL THAT IS RIGHT WITH ME

Sleep deprivation affects our mood. We can feel down and become irritable and snappy with people around us. In turn, this affects our thoughts, and we may become caught up in a cycle of judging and blaming ourselves or others. When we are caught up in a negative spiral like this, it's difficult to remember all the things that are actually okay in our lives.

This practice is about recognizing those things. You can do this as part of a formal sit, or informally at any time, including in bed.

## THE PRACTICE

1   If you are doing this practice as a formal meditation, check your posture (see page 58) and take a few moments to settle your attention on the breath. If you are doing it informally, simply check in with the breath before you start.

2   **Turn your attention to your body,** noticing and acknowledging the different parts:

- The legs that allow you to walk, run, and stand to watch the sun rise ...

- The arms that allow you to embrace loved ones, reach up for something on the top shelf, hang out the laundry ...

- The hands that allow you to stroke a pet, close buttons on your clothing, wash yourself in the shower ...

- The fingers and thumb that allow you to choose your favorite candy from the pack, thread a needle, pick up a pin from the floor ...

- The eyes that allow you to see someone you love, admire your friend's garden, watch your grandchild do a handstand ...

- The nose that allows you to breathe in the scent of honeysuckle or warns you that a food you were about to eat has gone bad ...

- The ears that allow you to hear the dawn chorus begin and crescendo while those around you are deaf to it ...

- The mouth that allows you to savor the taste of your favorite food ...

Continue in this way, choosing and acknowledging how different parts of your body allow you to enjoy your life in so many ways.

3 **Turn your attention to the people around you**—family, friends, neighbors, and coworkers. Take a moment to bring each one into your mind's eye, name them, and acknowledge what they bring to your life. Include those who take away the garbage each week, who look after you when you are sick, who serve you in the store ... Include any pets or animals in your life. Be as specific as you can. Continue in this way, choosing and acknowledging how many people contribute to the life you lead.

4 **Turn your attention to your environment**—your home, the neighborhood, the amenities, the parks ... Appreciate where you live.

5 **What else in your life can you take a moment to appreciate?**
Your place of work, a vacation, food to eat, clean water to drink, feeling safe ...

6 When you are ready, take a few moments to return your attention to the breath before finishing.

# AWAKE JUST LIKE ME

I once read about a woman who, in the early hours, tweeted about not being able to sleep and was immediately flooded with replies from fellow insomniacs. One of the frustrations of not sleeping is feeling that you are the only person awake (particularly if your partner is sleeping soundly next to you). In this practice we connect with the sense that we are never alone in our suffering, and that at any one time there will always be at least one other person experiencing something similar (although, in the case of insomnia, it is more likely to be hundreds of thousands, if not millions).

This practice is about connecting to others who are in a similar position to us. It is not about trying to fall asleep.

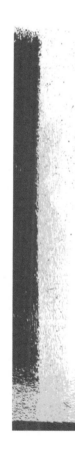

## THE PRACTICE

1   This can be done lying in bed. Begin by simply **becoming aware of the whole body**, noticing all the points where it is in contact with the bed. Lightly bring your attention to the breath, staying with the length of the in-breath, noticing that moment when an in-breath makes the transition to an out-breath, and then following the out-breath. Continue in this way, bringing the attention back whenever it wanders.

2   After a few minutes, expand your attention from the breath to include the whole body, becoming aware of **how it feels physically to be awake**. What are you experiencing? Notice how you may move toward some aspects of your experience that you like (such as a cool breeze touching warm skin), and pull back from those that you don't (perhaps tension in the shoulders). Notice any accompanying thoughts or emotions that may indicate how you are relating to whatever is arising. We are not searching for anything in

particular. **Whatever you are experiencing is your experience.** You may like to reassure yourself by saying silently, "It's okay, let me feel this."

3 Then **expand your attention to include others like you**, lying awake when they would rather be sleeping. If there is a friend or family member who you know is often in a similar position, bring him or her specifically to mind, otherwise imagine those in your immediate neighborhood who might be awake right now: insomniacs, a nursing mother, someone sick and in pain, the firefighter, nurse, physician, police officer, the person in the 24-hour grocery store, the truck driver delivering fresh produce … **each one of them awake, just like you**. You may like to hold the images of these different people in your mind one at a time and then wish them well. Further guidance on how you might bring these people to mind and the type of phrases you could use to send them your good wishes is given overleaf.

4 Conclude the practice by narrowing your attention back to the breath for a minute or two.

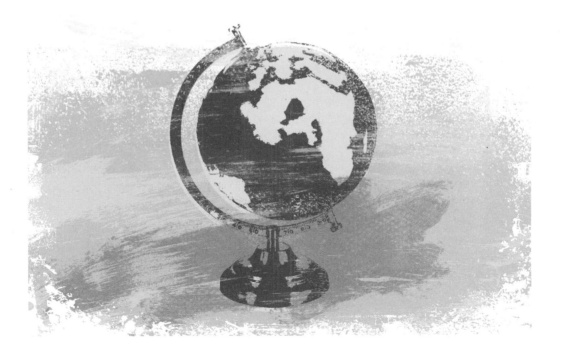

# WHO IS AWAKE JUST LIKE YOU?

As you think of those who are awake, just like you, use the words below for guidance.

When bringing to mind **a mother nursing a baby,**
silently repeat to yourself:
*Awake just like me: May you be well, may you be happy, may you feel rested.*

Adapt the words as you wish. **The exact words are less important than the intention to connect with others in the same position as you.**
Slowly repeat them a few times, simply offering them without any expectations. You are unlikely to feel anything in particular, and that is okay.

Then picture yourself with this person (or a generic image if it is not someone specific) and repeat:
*May we be well, may we be happy, may we feel rested.*

Now bring to mind **someone who is sick** and being kept awake by their pain:
*Awake just like me: May you be well, may you be happy,
may you feel rested (or variations).*

Repeat as before, and then include yourself with this person:
*May we be well, may we be happy, may we feel rested.*

Keep adding as many different types of person as you wish,
**including those whose jobs continue through the night in order to protect and serve others.**

Finally, you may like to offer these good wishes to
**everyone anywhere who is awake:**
*All those who are awake, just like me: May we be well, may we be happy,
may we feel rested.*

# WHAT NOURISHES YOU?

**If we are not sleepy, it will be impossible to fall asleep, and lying awake becoming frustrated is not helpful. Acknowledging and accepting that since we are awake we might as well be awake is a more helpful attitude. We can be awake and engage in an activity that feels positive and nourishing, or maybe one that gives us a sense of satisfaction.**

Some activities might be things you can do in bed, but it can be helpful to actually get up—since that reinforces the idea that we spend time in bed only if we are sleepy or sleeping. If you begin to feel sleepy as you do one of these activities, stop and go back to bed.

## NOURISHING ACTIVITIES

Take a moment to think about what nourishes you. Make a list, so you have something you can easily refer to. Here are some ideas to get you started:

- Reading
- Listening to music, a podcast, or an audiobook
- Playing a musical instrument (if you can do so without disturbing neighbors or others sleeping in the house!)
- Doing yoga stretches
- Meditating
- Knitting
- Making something
- Fixing a hot drink
- Cooking or preparing food
- Coloring in a coloring book
- Writing in a journal

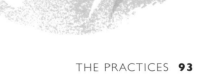

## SATISFYING ACTIVITIES

Take a moment to think about what activities you find satisfying, and what you could do without disturbing neighbors or others in the house. Make a list, so you have something you can easily refer to. Here are a few examples:

- Tidying—a desk, closet, or room
- Cleaning—either a room, or washing the dishes
- Ironing or sorting laundry
- Watering the garden (if you can do so at night) or houseplants
- Filing paperwork
- Making a food shopping list for the week
- Organizing books or DVDs
- Packing a bag or preparing your outfit for the following day

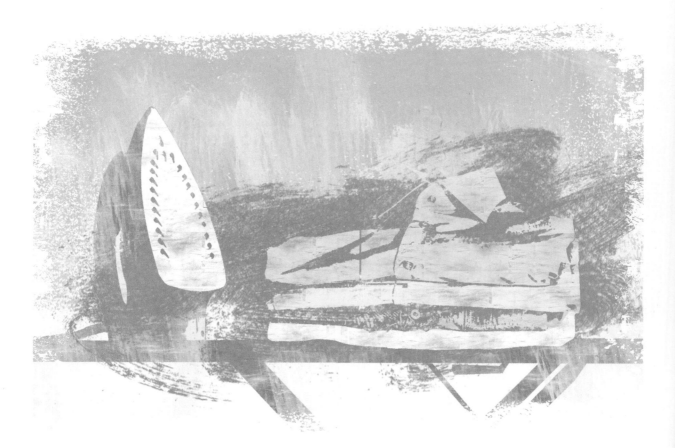

# WHAT IS YOUR BEDTIME STORY?

How we relate to being awake when we want to sleep determines the degree of suffering we experience. When we resist our experience and want it to be different, we are disappointed with the way things are. We may create mental stories about it, catastrophizing ("This is a nightmare"), generalizing ("I'm never able to sleep"), blaming ("This is all my fault—or someone else's"), crystal ball-gazing ("I'm not going to fall asleep" or "I'm going to be exhausted tomorrow"), judging ("I should be able to sleep"), and so on. We get so caught up in these stories that we believe them, but actually they are just a reflection of our state of mind.

The first step in breaking unhelpful cycles such as these is to become aware of them. Then we can choose how to respond to what we become aware of. We can't do anything differently until we know what is arising right now. Try it and see.

## NAMING THE MONSTERS

Notice what particular story is being played out in your head tonight. Simply notice and acknowledge it (no need to give yourself a hard time about it): "Ah, it's the 'This is all my fault' blockbuster tonight!"

The more we do this, the more we start to notice the same old tales appearing again and again. We can introduce a bit of humor and give each one a silly title. Naming the monsters is always a good way to undermine them and gain some perspective.

## YOUR PERCEIVED AMOUNT OF SLEEP

Once, after a broken night, I told a friend, "It was terrible—I was awake for hours." I felt exhausted. Yet when I looked at my fitness tracker, which has a sleep monitor, it had recorded 8½ hours' sleep. I laughed as I noticed that just reading that immediately made me feel better (despite knowing it wasn't that accurate): My perception had changed.

A word of caution about sleep monitors: They are not always accurate; mine, for example, which I use for exercise, says that I'm asleep when I'm meditating or reading (i.e. not moving). They can encourage us to focus too closely on how much or how little sleep we've had. It is healthier to become familiar with your body's own signals and respond when it feels tired or refreshed.

## BRINGING OUR ATTENTION INTO THE PRESENT MOMENT

We can redirect our attention to the breath in the belly or simply become aware of the body. We can be curious about any physical sensations arising internally and externally, perhaps noticing temperature or a draft on the skin. Bringing our attention to the body and its changing sensations shifts it out of the head and into the present moment.

## SHIFTING OUT OF THE HEAD INTO THE BODY

We can also notice how the story is manifesting in the body, since negative stories often generate tension and uncomfortable sensations. Notice how it makes you feel physically and emotionally. Bring a friendly interest to whatever you notice, and remind yourself that there is no need to do anything to fix or change what you become aware of.

# KEEPING THE TIGERS AWAY

**There is a wonderful Sufi teaching story about being unaware of how our patterns of behavior affect us.**

The story is about a man who scattered crumbs around his house each night. A curious neighbor asked him what he was doing. "I'm keeping the tigers away," he replied.

"But there are no tigers around here," the neighbor said.

"Exactly!" replied the man triumphantly.

We often fall into patterns of behavior that are supposed to be helpful, but can end up being very restrictive. We believe that if we do this, this, and that, then we will be able to sleep—and sometimes we do, which simply reinforces the pattern. However, inevitably there are conditions and circumstances that we can't control, and when these aren't just so it creates additional anxiety. The more flexibility we can develop in our routines, the easier we will find it when things are not quite as we would like them to be.

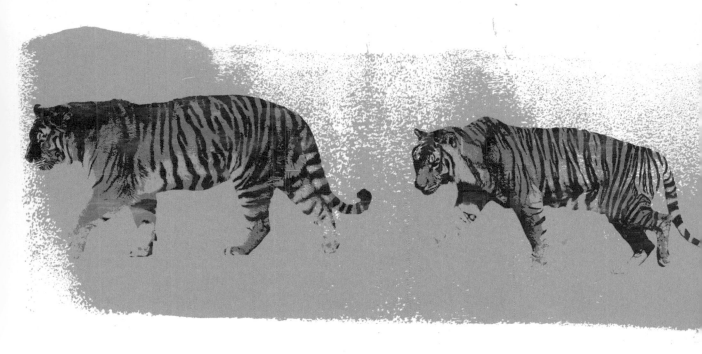

# THE PRACTICE

1   What routines do you employ to "keep the tigers away"? Checking the clock in the night? Counting the number of hours you did or didn't sleep? Working out how often you woke up in the night? Working out how many hours' sleep you might still be able to get? Checking the temperature of the room? Performing a going-to-bed sequence in a particular order? **Imagine letting just one of these go, or doing it differently.** As you bring that thought to mind, become aware of how it feels in the head (thoughts), heart (emotions), and body (physical sensations). What do you notice?

2   Run through all your routines and notice if any generates a stronger response than the others. Which has the weakest response? If we notice an unwillingness to let something go, it suggests that **we are too strongly attached to it.** Holding on to something too tightly takes effort and makes us fear what might happen if it wasn't there. We often catastrophize and imagine the worst possible scenario. Just notice that to begin with.

3   Choose the routine that generated the weakest response, and, if you are willing to give it a go, **experiment with doing it differently.** You could even drop it entirely. Be as creative as you can. Approach it as an experiment, remaining open to the outcome. Have no expectations. Continue for a few days with that particular routine, and when you feel ready, choose another. Experiment with that for a short time, then choose another, and so on.

4   Be patient with yourself, and **move at a pace that feels comfortable.** You may want to have breaks every so often, when you leave things as they are for a while. There is no rush, and it is always your choice.

5   Cultivate a sense of curiosity and play. **Notice how you feel in the head, heart, and body** in anticipation of doing something differently, then as you are doing it, and then reflect afterward.

   If it feels too difficult to begin with routines connected to sleep, start with the practice on the opposite page, Out of the Ordinary.

# OUT OF THE ORDINARY

**The previous exercise might feel too much to begin with. Sometimes it is easier to begin by changing activities that are unconnected to sleep. We can start to build up flexibility and a willingness to do something differently during the day, with activities that are less emotionally charged than our sleep routines.**

When we do something that is very closely tied to routine, we are operating on autopilot. When we are on autopilot, it is as if we are sleepwalking. We are unaware of our surroundings, we have no awareness of what we are doing, and we are often wrapped up in our thoughts to the exclusion of all else. However, when we do something out of the ordinary we wake up, and the body instinctively becomes alert—something new is happening! Our senses become more acute and our experience becomes sharper and more memorable. It's not about making the experience more positive—although often it can feel more enjoyable—but about being willing to step outside of our comfort zone and do something differently.

Use your imagination and come up with something you can do each day that is out of the ordinary. Wake yourself up!

## TRY THESE

- Take a different route to work, the store, or school with the kids.
- Choose a different food for lunch and eat it in a different place from normal.
- Learn something new—a craft, a language, a musical instrument, how to put up a shelf or plant some herbs …
- Talk to the person who is serving you in the store or cafe.
- Try a food you have never tasted before.
- Try a food or drink that you always say you dislike.
- If you go to a class or regular meeting, sit in a different place.

# BREAKING THE TYRANNY OF TECHNOLOGY

The negative impact of technology on our sleep can be significant (see page 24), but we may not be aware of how insidious our use has become. Checking our smartphones can become so habitual that often we don't even realize we are doing it. This practice offers an opportunity to explore how you use technology and whether it rules you, rather than vice versa, and to discover more about how it affects you personally.

It is essential with any exploration of this kind that you engage with an attitude of curiosity and interest. Whatever you discover counts as feedback—and, if you wish, an opportunity to begin doing something differently—rather than harsh judgment.

## KEEP A RECORD

Start by simply beginning to track what you are doing. Ideally, keep this record over several days, paying particular attention to your habits in the evenings. (If you have created a sleep diary (see Chapter 4), you could use it to record this information.)

Make notes about the device(s):

- What are you using? Television, laptop, tablet, e-reader, and/or smartphone.
- When are you using each one? Notice particularly what is the last device you use before bed, and at what time you turn it off in relation to going to bed.
- How long are you using each one?

Make notes about your sleep:

- What time do you go to bed?
- What time do you fall asleep? (Record this the next day.)
- What time do you wake up?
- How was your quality of sleep?

Make notes about your day (both before and after using the device):

- What do you notice about your attention and focus?
- What do you notice about your mood?
- What do you notice about your energy level?

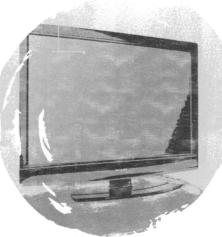

Alongside making these notes, try the following practice to help you notice your experience. It may be too much to pay attention to all your devices at any one time, so you can always choose one, perhaps the one you use the most just before bedtime.

## THE PRACTICE

1 Begin **noticing the impulse to turn on the device.** What happens just before? How do you feel, both physically and mentally? For example, with the television, perhaps you are feeling exhausted and just want to zone out in front of it, or maybe you are keen to watch something specific that interests you. Perhaps you are bored … Simply notice.

2 How do you feel during and after the activity? Do you feel nourished, refreshed, and invigorated, or depleted and drained?

3 Notice **whether you would have done something else** if you hadn't been bingeing on a box set or watching cats do silly things on YouTube. What would that activity have been, and how does it compare with what you actually did? Do you check your smartphone when you are talking or listening to someone else? How does it feel when someone does that to you? How about when you are having a meal? How does divided attention affect your experience of eating in terms of noticing flavor, texture, and when you have had enough?

# NEXT STEPS

Once you have built up a picture of whether your use of technological devices is out of kilter or not, you may decide to do something differently, such as limiting a particular device at certain times. If you do this, notice how it feels in the head (thoughts), heart (emotions), and body (physical sensations), checking in with yourself at the start of the period of abstinence and then periodically during it. If there are moments of anxiety or even panic, drop your attention to your feet on the floor and, concentrating on your breath, imagine that you are breathing in and out through the soles of your feet (see page 67).

You may decide to go "cold turkey," but this is an experiment, so you have control over how long a period of abstinence you want to try. If your habits are strong, start with shorter periods and build up to longer, ideally working back from your bedtime. It is recommended that you have a minimum of one hour without using a device before you plan to go to sleep, but we are all different, so in the first instance explore what is helpful for you (see page 100). It can help to plan alternative activities to engage in for longer periods of abstinence from technology.

Notice over a period of time—ideally several days—how changing these automatic patterns of behavior affects your mood, habits, and sleep. Remember to let go of any particular expectations: The success of any experiment relies on maintaining an open mind about the results.

## EXPERIMENTING AS A FAMILY

Children often copy what their parents do, so unhelpful habits with technology will probably show up in all family members, and children will be as adversely affected as adults by the misuse of devices (see page 25). Experiment with the above practice involving all family members, making it fun and engaging rather than punitive. You can use charts and rewards suitable for the children's ages. Think about what activities you can do instead—reading a bedtime story, asking about one another's days, playing a game … Be creative, and use the experiment as an opportunity to strengthen your relationships with one another.

Before you order your children to turn off the television, and confiscate their smartphones while you are secretly checking your emails, consider whether it's fair to ask something of them that you are not prepared to do yourself.

# EXPLORING RESISTANCE

**Suffering is often the result of resisting our experience. We don't like the way we are, the way someone else is, or a particular situation, and we wish things were different. Resisting the way things actually are generates a lot of physical tension in the body (as we brace ourselves against what is arising), as well as mental exhaustion (as we try to fix or change what is arising).**

If you have trouble sleeping, you will have experienced something like this as you lie in bed. You may feel physically tired, but you are awake and your mind is hyper-alert—worrying about not sleeping, wondering why, thinking about the next day and how you are going to feel more exhausted, and so on and so on. We can feel stuck, going round and round like a hamster on a wheel, and we don't know how to step out of it.

We can't do anything about feeling physically tired; that is how the body is right now. We can, however, do something about all the additional layers of suffering we are adding on top of "body tired"—the thoughts about not sleeping and its consequences. That is within our control. Resisting how things are is the problem, therefore the easiest way to relax or let go is to stop trying to make things different.

Whenever we are learning new skills, it is better to begin with something minor that doesn't have a strong emotional charge—perhaps something that has nothing to do with sleep. It could be a moment during an unpleasant commute, feeling frustrated as you stand in line when you are in a rush, or when you are late for an appointment and you are being held up in traffic.

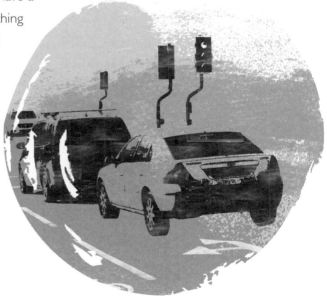

# THE PRACTICE

1　First of all, **be aware that things are not as you would like them to be**. This is easier to pick up if you have been doing a body-focused practice such as Paying Attention to the Breath (see page 61), Paying Attention to the Body (see page 71), or the Body Scan (see page 68) regularly, since usually the first signs we notice are those arising from the body. Perhaps there is tension in the neck or shoulders, maybe we are tapping our feet, drumming our fingers, or clenching our jaw … each person has their own physical signs of stress.

2　Once you are aware, **acknowledge it, saying "Resistance is here"** (or words to that effect, such as "Irritation is here"). Acknowledging and naming what is here is the first step toward accepting it.

3　Then **tune in to how that resistance or emotion feels in the body**. Where are you feeling it? How does it feel: Solid or soft? Is it moving or staying in one place? Are there any sensations associated with it (tingling, pulsing, stabbing …)? Be curious about how resistance actually feels. If there are no strong sensations but just a sense of numbness, that is equally interesting: How far does the numbness extend around the body? What can you discover?

4　We are not trying to make the resistance or emotion go away. We are **exploring how it feels to be with it**—to **allow it to be present**, since it already is. You could say silently to yourself, "It's okay, let me feel this."

5　We may stay with the physical sensations of the resistance only fleetingly before taking our attention to the breath or breathing through the feet on the floor to anchor ourselves. We may choose to dip back and forth between the breath and the sensations, but only if it feels okay to do so. Stay with the uncomfortable sensations for a brief period only when you begin to do this.

6 There is nothing to be gained by gritting your teeth determinedly. It is important to **explore gently and with a strong sense of kindness.** If your attention is pulled away from the body by thoughts about what is arising, simply acknowledge those thoughts and redirect your attention to the body or the breath.

7 You don't need to spend very long doing this practice informally as you go about your day. It can take just a couple of minutes.

8 Experiment with this informal practice. Begin with life's small irritations, and, when you have some experience and feel comfortable doing that, experiment with how it feels when you are lying awake. It is very important to **let go of wanting to fix or change your experience**, since that is counterproductive. This practice is about **learning to accept things as they are**—even when we don't like them.

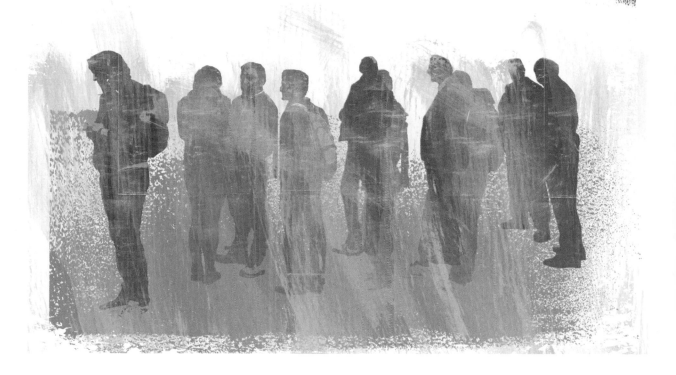

# EXPLORING THE SENSES

All mindfulness practices are about facilitating that shift from "doing" to "being" mode. A simple way to do this is to use our senses. We can do this practice when we are out and about, at home, or lying in bed.

Notice how you relate to whatever arises. Do you like it? Do you dislike it? Are you neutral? Just become aware, and be willing to stay with any sense and see what arises. Things may emerge that you miss at first.

## THE PRACTICE

1  **SIGHT:** What is in your line of vision right now? Perhaps **notice the colors**—how light affects a color so that it becomes more than just a hue. Notice how it is made up of multiple tones and even includes different colors. How many different shades of white can you see? How many different colors can you see within white? Name them.

   When you are ready, let go of Sight and move your attention to Sound.

2  **SOUND:** Imagine that **the body is a radar** picking up any sound that comes its way. Each sound is made up of a collection of notes; some make pleasing combinations, but others are more strident and unpleasant. Notice whether there is **a physical response to a sound**. If you find yourself creating a story about a sound, acknowledge it and let it go. We are simply tuning into the music of the universe right now.

   When you are ready, let go of Sound and move your attention to Smell.

3 **SMELL:** Take a deep breath in through the nose. What do you notice? Continue to breathe in and **explore scents and smells**, liking, not liking, and indifference.

When you are ready, let go of Smell and move your attention to Taste.

4 **TASTE:** Become aware of any lingering taste or flavor in the mouth—is there a hint of something? Maybe not. Simply explore, **without any expectation of finding anything**.

When you are ready, let go of Taste and move your attention to Touch.

5 **TOUCH:** Become aware of the different textures in contact with your skin. **How do they feel?** How many can you name? We may experience the touch of objects or clothing, or perhaps the environment—a cold draft against the skin. Become aware of how they may change or of others that come and go …

6 Finish by taking a moment to become **aware of the body as a whole**.

# IT'S OKAY, I'M OKAY

When we are anxious, the body's internal threat system is activated. Stress hormones, including adrenaline, noradrenaline, and cortisol, are released, and the body moves into a state of hyper-vigilance—we are wired for action. All this undermines the state of mind needed for sleep. We can, however, reassure ourselves that we are okay and, by doing so, turn off the body's alarm system.

As with many of the practices in this book, this one can be done when lying in bed, but also at any point during the day. We are bringing our helpful attitudes (see pages 50–52) to this practice, including non-striving, curiosity, and kindness.

## MINDFULNESS AND ANXIETY

Many people suffer from anxiety: According to AnxietyUK, it is around 5 people in every 100 in the UK, and it's more likely to affect women than men. Unlike stress, where there is often a specific external trigger such as work, illness, or relationships, the cause of anxiety is less specific, and often the sufferer won't know why they feel the way they do. When we are anxious about something, the body's internal threat system is repeatedly (and needlessly) activated, with a range of physical and psychological consequences.

Mindfulness is one way of learning to manage the condition. Through it, we learn to spot the unhelpful story, pick up the physical manifestation in the body, and practice grounding techniques such as focusing on the breath or breathing through the feet on the floor. By doing this we learn to move toward and "be" with what is arising, rather than avoiding it—and, paradoxically, this changes our relationship with it, making it easier and less frightening. A review of the research into mindfulness and anxiety by Hofmann, Sawyer, Witt, and Oh (2010) of 39 studies of mindfulness-based therapy for a range of conditions, including anxiety, found that mindfulness was a "promising intervention" for treating anxiety and problems with mood.

# THE PRACTICE

1   Begin by becoming aware of the whole body in contact with the surface.
Notice any points of contact and that sense of weight as the body softens
into the mattress. You may want to place a hand on your belly or over your
collarbone so the tips of the fingers are at the base of the neck (and you can
feel the pulse in the neck). Start **tuning in to the sensations arising
in the body**: The belly rising and falling as breath enters and leaves the body;
the flutter against the fingertips that is the heart beating.

2   Check in with yourself, asking "What's going on for me right now?" Turn to
the **head** (thoughts), **heart** (emotions), and **body** (physical sensations), and
notice what, if anything, is present. Name it—for example "Anxiety is here,"
"Butterflies in the stomach," and so on. Then return your attention to the
breath and the body, really connecting to any felt sensations.

3   Begin saying silently to yourself, **"It's okay, I'm okay."** You can repeat one
statement on each in-breath and the other on each out-breath. It is important
to acknowledge that in this moment you are okay. You may be awake and you
may be anxious, but **in this moment you are safe and breathing**.

4   Continue self-soothing in this way, using these phrases or others of your
own. We are soothing ourselves in the same way that we would **comfort
a distressed child**, reassuring them, repeating the words over and over.
The hand on the belly or the top of the chest reinforces that sense of
connection with the body. Whenever the attention wanders, bring it back
without any judgment.

5   Continue for as long as you wish, remembering that **there is no
expectation that your experience will change**. The feeling
of anxiety may continue, or you may notice that it changes in some way.
Approach the practice with the open mind of a scientist performing an
experiment for the very first time, without any knowledge or expectation
of what might arise.

# IDENTIFYING AND TACKLING STRESS

Feeling overwhelmed and unable to cope with what we are facing causes us to feel stressed. When we are stressed, the body's threat or stress reaction is activated and the body prepares to battle the perceived threat (see page 46). This reaction is activated by the amygdala, the most primitive part of the brain. The more frequently the amygdala is activated, the more sensitive it becomes. As a survival mechanism it works brilliantly, but evolution hasn't caught up with the modern world, so these days it is usually activated by situations that are anything but life or death.

Having trouble sleeping is often a sign that we are stressed. By doing before-and-after scans, neuroscientists discovered that eight weeks of mindfulness training with regular home practice led to a decrease in the activation of the amygdala, meaning that people were feeling less stressed. Mindfulness can help with stress because it activates the body's in-built calming response. In addition, through practicing we become used to tuning in to the body and picking up early signs that we are feeling stressed, and we can take wise action to nip it in the bud.

## WHAT ARE YOUR STRESS INDICATORS?

These indicators are different for each one of us, so it is worth becoming familiar with yours. Take a moment to reflect on the following questions.

**What makes you stressed?** Cast your mind back to incidents that you perceived as stressful and that perhaps affected your sleep. What were they? You may notice patterns involving particular situations, people, and places. Just notice these for future reference. This is about becoming familiar with your own vulnerabilities so that you can take care of yourself, and it is important not to fall into the trap of anticipating that because one particular thing happened you will feel stressed, or not sleep. Always cultivate beginner's mind (see page 51).

**Where in the body do you feel it physically when you are stressed?** Common places are the belly—a twisted feeling in the gut, perhaps—the neck and shoulders (tension and stiffness), and the jaw (grinding your teeth in the night is a common sign of stress). However, there could be other places in the body where you feel physical discomfort when you are stressed. Be as specific as you can and make a note of them. If you are not sure, start paying attention to the body next time you feel stressed, and notice what arises. Some sensations will be "in the moment," whereas others will be the result of tension that builds up over time.

**How does stress affect your behavior and frame of mind?** Feeling irritable or short-tempered is a common reaction. We may find that we drink more alcohol or caffeine, or eat less healthily. Some people eat more; others eat less. Disrupted sleep is also a common side effect. Be as honest as you can when making this list. The purpose is to highlight indicators that can serve as red flags for you in the future. We can't change our behavior until we are aware of it.

**How could you take care of yourself when you are feeling stressed?** It's helpful to build up a repertoire of activities that you know will help you when you are stressed. Here are some examples:

- If you are at work, take time away from your desk for lunch (rather than eating while working or even skipping it altogether), go to chat to a coworker, or take a moment to look out the window.
- Focus on the breath for a moment or two to help you to pause.
- Do a high-intensity activity to help to dispel stress hormones from the body.
- Take a soothing hot candlelit bath with gentle music playing, or go out for an evening walk, to make you feel calmer.
- Do a body-focused practice if your mind is particularly busy.
- Make something—a tasty meal or a knitting, crochet, or other craft project.
- Gain a wider perspective by spending time with others, but be careful of rehashing the stressful situation over and over, since that can keep fueling the fire of stress.

Start paying attention to what you find helpful, and make a note of it so that you can refer to it in difficult moments.

# THE IMPORTANCE OF EXERCISE

**If we are feeling fatigued through not sleeping, the last thing we probably feel like doing is exercise. However, exercising the body will make us feel physically tired, as well as lift our mood and improve our overall health.**

Research into mindfulness and sleep (see page 53) includes an element of gentle stretching, and participants often remark that it is beneficial. If we are feeling stressed, a brisk walk, run, or swim can help to disperse stress hormones such as adrenaline, which can keep us in a state of arousal.

## WHAT EXERCISE DO YOU DO AT THE MOMENT?

Take a minute to reflect and write down what you already do. This might include walking to the store or with the children to school, or perhaps you are on your feet all day at home or at work. Include any form of movement that you do in your day. You might do more than you think.

However, if you find that you do very little exercise or if you would simply like to do more, start to think about what you could do. What is stopping you? Notice any thoughts that arise. Explore the resistance if it feels particularly strong. It is always better to start small and build up your capacity gradually—just adding a few extra steps a day can set you on the right path. The various digital trackers that count steps and other activity can be a good incentive.

Many activities can be adapted if you have limited mobility (yoga is a particularly good example), but always discuss your needs with an experienced practitioner. It's important that any exercise is suitable for your age and health. If you haven't exercised for a while and you have health problems, do consult your physician first.

Exercising outside has the added benefit of allowing you to get a dose of fresh air and connect with the natural world.

Remember that it can be counterproductive to exercise too close to going to bed, since a raised body temperature will interfere with the body's natural sleep systems. If possible, always leave at least 3 hours to cool down before bedtime.

## EXERCISE YOU COULD TRY

- Swimming
- Walking
- Tai chi
- Qigong
- Running
- Yoga
- Pilates
- Cycling
- Dancing
- Spinning
- Gardening
- Ball games (tennis, badminton, netball, baseball, cricket, football, squash)

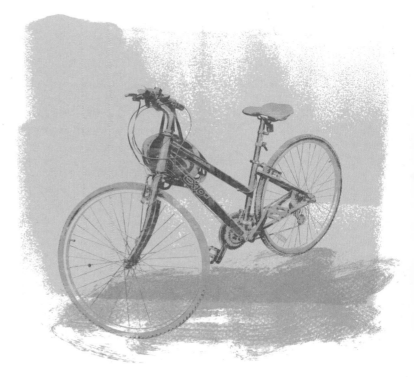

## OTHER IDEAS

- Take an exercise class—not only will you learn a new skill, but also it will encourage and support you, and it's an opportunity to meet new people.
- Park the car further from your destination, or get off the bus or train a stop early, so that you incorporate walking into your journey.
- Take the stairs or walk up an escalator.
- Give the dog an extra walk—if you don't have one, could you borrow one from a neighbor?
- Walk around the block.

# EXERCISING MINDFULLY

Exercising can be a great opportunity to integrate mindfulness into your everyday life. Any activity can be done mindfully, and the underlying principle is always to know what you are doing while you are doing it.

The following description of how to approach this is for running, but the principles are the same for any activity.

## Be aware of how it feels in the body.

- **Notice your breathing**—is it fast, slow, or labored? Are you holding your breath, perhaps? Notice how you respond to whatever you notice. If your breathing is labored, the story might include some self-judgment ("I'm so unfit") or perhaps anxiety ("I'm going to have a heart attack!"). The instruction is always just to notice the story and how it feels in the body. Staying as grounded as possible in the physical sensations of the body will help to prevent unhelpful thoughts from spiraling out of control. Remember that it is okay to stop and rest, and it is important that you do so if you feel unwell.
- **Notice your posture**, paying particular attention to any areas of tightness or tension. Are your shoulders raised? Are your hands clenched, or your jaw? Simply notice how the body reflects your state of mind. There is no need to actively try to change what you notice, although often when we become aware of tension—say in the shoulders—it will release naturally.
- **Notice the physical sensations of running**—the feet in contact with the ground. Which part of the foot makes contact first? What follows? Remember, we are not thinking about the action of running, but simply noticing it.

Scan through the whole body from time to time.

## Notice what is going on in the mind. Your body may be running through the park on a beautiful morning, but is your head already at work? When you notice that your attention is pulled away from the present moment (even by positive things), just bring it back to noticing the moment and what is arising internally as well as in the environment.

**Become aware of any emotions**—frustration, peace, calm, disappointment—name them, and be curious about whether there are accompanying, connected sensations in the body.

**Expand your awareness to include the environment around you**—the sights, sounds, and smells—from time to time. Drink them in. Notice which ones you are drawn to and which you recoil from. Can you identify a sense of liking or not liking in the body? Where does it manifest? How does it feel? Be as specific as you can.

These instructions are not a step-by-step sequence. All you need to remember is to check in to the head (thoughts), heart (emotions), and body (physical sensations) regularly throughout the activity, and notice what is arising.

It is also useful to notice what attitude you are bringing to the activity. Does it have a driven quality? A sign of this might be if you are focused on how fast or how far you have run, or how many calories you are burning. When we do something mindfully we are more interested in what we are experiencing in each moment than in an end goal.

This often means that we relax; paradoxically, this can improve performance, but that is not the aim.

When we are working out with other people, it can be interesting to notice whether our comparing mind kicks in—are we faster, slower, fitter, thinner, fatter than the person next to us? We may be judging ourselves or someone else, but either way, the invitation is simply to notice the thought—"There I go again"—and bring the attention back to the body and any physical sensations that may be arising. Practice non-judging of yourself and others and refresh the helpful attitudes on pages 50–52.

## EXERCISING WITH OTHERS

It is easier to exercise mindfully by ourselves, simply because we can focus exclusively on our own experience. If you are running and chatting with friends, for example, all your focus will be on that interaction. There is nothing wrong with this, and exercising with friends is a great way to support one another as well as to have fun. However, you may want to choose to do the activity on your own from time to time, so that you can practice it mindfully, or—if you are with others— just practice mindful awareness for a few minutes every so often.

Some types of class, for example a high-impact aerobics or spinning class, will be more challenging because of the pace, but you could still experiment with tuning in to the head, heart, and body from time to time, or even just before and after the class, and reflecting on your underlying intention and attitudes.

## BE CREATIVE

Be as creative as possible in the way you integrate mindfulness into your exercise routine. Focus on staying present as best you can, and consciously cultivate the attitudes described on pages 50–52. It is important to remember that exercising mindfully doesn't mean you will or must enjoy it. We are not trying to transform our experience; we are simply noticing how it is.

## OUR FRAME OF MIND CAN TRANSFORM AN EXPERIENCE

Some years ago I was persuaded to enter a 10km (6 mile) trail race. I was used to running in a flat city park and I had no experience of running across country. I mistakenly assumed that it would be just like running around the park. The race started badly—I was caught up with other runners, and the pace was too fast for me. Gradually I fell so far back that the next race, which was canicross (running with your dog), caught up with me, and as I stumbled along the trail with baying dogs at my heels I was not in a good place. Although I finished, I ran the entire race wishing I were somewhere else and cursing every step—total avoidance state of mind.

Despite swearing that I would never do anything like that again, I allowed myself to be persuaded, and less than a month later I found myself at another 10km start line. This time I had decided to run more mindfully. I hung back to let the pack get ahead, and I ran at my own pace. I enjoyed the sun on my face and being outside, drinking in the sights and smells. I paid attention to my posture, regularly scanning and noticing areas of tightness, particularly in my shoulders and neck, which caused them to release naturally. I let go of any expectations of achieving a time or place, and was happy just to complete the race. Although I wasn't much faster than I had been in the first race, the experience was vastly different. As I crossed the line someone asked me if I had enjoyed it and I realized that I had. I hadn't done any extra training—the only difference was my frame of mind. By consciously cultivating an approach state of mind and letting go of striving, I focused on the present moment. My mind was relaxed and so were the muscles in my body, and I experienced virtually no stiffness the following day, unlike after the first race.

If you are interested in a mindful approach to running, have a look at Danny Dreyer's Chi Running (www.chirunning.com).

# CHAPTER 4
# YOUR SLEEP DIARY

Here you will find instructions for keeping a sleep diary and pages where you can record what you notice about your habits and behavior, as you begin exploring what affects your sleep.

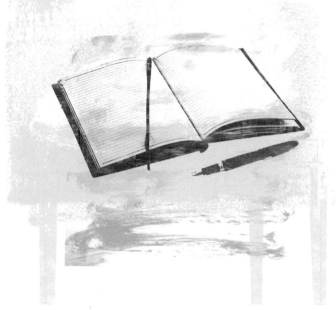

# HOW TO KEEP A SLEEP DIARY

**It's useful to keep a note of what we discover once we start paying attention to our routine and behavior and noticing how that affects our sleep, whether positively or negatively. You can either photocopy the diary pages on 124–125 or just jot things down in a notebook.**

We have included examples of filled-in pages on pages 122–123 to give you an idea of the kind of thing you might record in your sleep diary. You might want to note what is happening for you at work or home, if you are working extra hours or doing shift work, and if you are traveling, particularly across time zones. It's fine to estimate times and amounts for awakenings and activities, and for food and drink consumption.

In the review section, note any insights into what may be helping or hindering your sleep. If you start implementing new positive habits (see page 36), make a note of what they are and what you notice. Small changes make a difference, so alter one thing at a time and continue it for at least a couple of weeks.

The aim of the sleep diary is to give you an insight into what you could do to help yourself. Generally, when we become aware of unhelpful habits we naturally begin to change them. However, it is important not to become fixated on doing things in a particular way. If you find that keeping notes increases your anxiety, perhaps set them aside for a while. Practicing mindfulness encourages flexibility and a willingness to be with the way things are, so in time you may find it helpful to go back to trying a sleep diary if you would like to.

## REMEMBER HELPFUL ATTITUDES

Keeping a sleep diary is an opportunity to continue this experiment with yourself as the object of study. Therefore, I would encourage you to consciously bring to mind the key pillars of mindfulness practice:

- **Be honest** It's easy to discount that extra glass of wine you had, and not record it, but acknowledging the way things really are (rather than the way we would like them to be) is at the heart of mindfulness. What you record is for your eyes only, and remember, you can't make any positive changes until you know where you are really starting from.

- **Be curious rather than judgmental** There's no need to be critical of anything you notice; simply notice cause and effect.

- **Be gentle with yourself** If you have a day when you slip back into unhelpful habits, just notice how they affect your sleep, rather than giving yourself a hard time. Noticing how we talk to ourselves when things don't go to plan, and practicing self-compassion, is as much a mindfulness practice as meditating for 15 minutes.

- **Let go of striving for a particular outcome** This will always be a challenge when you are recording something with a view to seeing an improvement, but with any experiment it is best to keep an open mind and let go of the desire for a particular outcome, which might blind us to the unexpected. I'd encourage you to notice when that sense of striving or disappointment arises if things don't turn out as you expect. Notice the thoughts, emotions, and physical sensations in the body and tune in to the breath for a few rounds, perhaps reassuring yourself at the same time, reminding yourself "It's okay." You can support non-striving by deciding to record for a period of time (say a week) before reviewing the data you've collected. Then continue for another period of time before reviewing once more.

- **Be patient** Remember, change takes time and it's rarely linear—there will be good days and nights, and those that are less good. When we experience the latter, it doesn't mean that everything we have been doing has been worthless. It's just the way things are.

I would suggest keeping a sleep diary for a specific period of time (at least 2 weeks) so that you can build up a picture of which habits are helpful for you and which are not. Once you are familiar with those, let go of the need to record how much sleep you have had or not. It's similar to the way weighing ourselves every day can be counterproductive, since we often start obsessing about minor changes up and down. The less anxious we are about how much sleep we are getting, the more likely we are to feel more relaxed—and that is conducive to feeling rested and refreshed and possibly sleeping better.

# EXAMPLE DIARY PAGES

## COMPLETE IN THE MORNING

I went to bed at: **10.30** AM / PM

I got up at: **6.30** AM / PM

Last night I fell asleep: Easily / After some time / With difficulty

I woke up: **About 4** times

Durations: **Once for about half an hour, for the other times just a few minutes**

I was disturbed by: Worry / Stress / Noise / Pain / Light

Other:

I slept a total of: **About 6 and half** hours

When I woke up I felt: Refreshed / Okay / Tired

Any other observations? **It was after a bad dream.**
**It took a while to get back to sleep.**

Review: Note any insights into what may be helping or hindering your sleep. **I was working right up to before I went to bed so then I couldn't sleep because my mind was full of all sorts of thoughts. I couldn't switch off!**

## COMPLETE AT THE END OF THE DAY

I took a nap:

Yes / No

Time: ........................................................... AM / PM

Duration: ...........................................................

During the day I felt:

Refreshed / Okay / Tired

Today my mood was:

Okay, a bit irritable

**Exercise**
List type/time/duration

Walked to and from work, about
40 minutes overall

**Alcohol consumption**
List type/time/amount

1 glass of red wine after evening meal

**Caffeine consumption**
List type/time/amount

3 cups of coffee 10 AM, 11.30 AM, 3 PM

**Heavy meals**
List type/time

Evening meal, 7.30 PM

**Medications**
List type/time

None

Describe activities in the hour
before bedtime including television,
computer/tablet/e-reader/cellphone
use, socializing, exercise, etc.

I was using my cellphone for about half an hour in
bed before trying to get to sleep.

Review: Note any insights into
what may be helping or hindering
your sleep.

Despite feeling really tired all day, I couldn't sleep
when I wanted to. I was trying to distract my
mind by playing on my cellphone but I think it
made me more awake.

# MY SLEEP DIARY

DATE:     /     /                    COMPLETE IN THE MORNING

I went to bed at: ............................................................................................ AM / PM

I got up at: ............................................................................................ AM / PM

Last night I fell asleep:    Easily / After some time / With difficulty

I woke up: ............................................................................................ times

Durations: ............................................................................................
............................................................................................

I was disturbed by:    Worry / Stress / Noise / Pain / Light

Other: ............................................................................................
............................................................................................
............................................................................................

I slept a total of: ............................................................................................ hours

When I woke up I felt:    Refreshed / Okay / Tired

Any other observations? ............................................................................................
............................................................................................
............................................................................................

Review: Note any insights
into what may be helping
or hindering your sleep.
............................................................................................
............................................................................................
............................................................................................

## COMPLETE AT THE END OF THE DAY

I took a nap

Yes / No

Time: ...........................................................................

Duration: .....................................................................

During the day I felt:

Refreshed / Okay / Tired

Today my mood was:

.........................................................................................

**Exercise**

List type/time/duration

.........................................................................................

.........................................................................................

**Alcohol consumption**

List type/time/amount

.........................................................................................

.........................................................................................

**Caffeine consumption**

List type/time/amount

.........................................................................................

.........................................................................................

**Heavy meals**

List type/time

.........................................................................................

.........................................................................................

**Medications**

List type/time

.........................................................................................

.........................................................................................

Describe activities in the hour
before bedtime including television,
computer/tablet/e-reader/cellphone
use, socializing, exercise, etc.

.........................................................................................

.........................................................................................

.........................................................................................

.........................................................................................

Review: Note any insights into
what may be helping or hindering
your sleep.

.........................................................................................

.........................................................................................

.........................................................................................

# INDEX

# RESOURCES

The following websites are useful sources of information for mindfulness courses and finding registered teachers in the UK and USA.

## CENTRE FOR MINDFULNESS PRACTICE AND RESEARCH (UK)

www.bangor.ac.uk/mindfulness

## OXFORD MINDFULNESS CENTRE (UK)

www.oxfordmindfulness.org

## BE MINDFUL (UK)

Search for courses near you; this site also offers online courses.
www.bemindful.co.uk

## UK NETWORK FOR MINDFULNESS-BASED TEACHER TRAINING ORGANIZATIONS

This has a listing of professional teachers who have shown that they meet the UK Good Practice Guidance for Mindfulness-based teachers.
www.mindfulnessteachersuk.org.uk/uk-listing

## CENTER FOR MINDFULNESS IN MEDICINE, HEALTH CARE, AND SOCIETY (USA)

www.umassmed.edu/cfm

# ACKNOWLEDGMENTS

I'd like to thank the following people at CICO Books: Cindy Richards for starting the conversation about mindfulness and sleep, Carmel Edmonds for her calm guidance throughout the process, Clare Nicholas for her terrific illustrations, and all those working tirelessly behind the scenes: Rosie Fairhead, Emily Breen, Sally Powell, Gordana Simakovic, Penny Craig, Kristine Pidkameny, and Dawn Bates, as well as those others whom I am not aware of!